About the Authors

Michael Kidd, AM, is the Executive Dean of the Faculty of Health Sciences at Flinders University and works as a general practitioner in an inner-city suburb. He was president of the Royal Australian College of General Practitioners from 2002 to 2006. He is president-elect of the World Organization of Family Doctors.

Leanne Rowe, AM, is a general practitioner and Deputy Chancellor of Monash University. She is a former Chairman of the Royal Australian College of General Practitioners and serves on the boards of Medibank Private and *beyondblue*. She is a past recipient of the 'Best Contribution to Health Care in Australia' awarded by the Australian Medical Association.

This edition published in 2011
First published in 2007

Arena, an imprint of Allen & Unwin
83 Alexander Street
Crows Nest NSW 2065
Australia
Phone: (61 2) 8425 0100
Fax: (61 2) 9906 2218
Email: info@allenandunwin.com
Web: www.allenandunwin.com

Cataloguing-in-publication details are available from the National Library of Australia: www.librariesaustralia.nla.gov.au

ISBN 978 1 74237 693 6

Text design by Christine Schiedel
Set in 10.5/13.5 pt Meta Plus by Midland Typesetters, Australia
Printed in Australia by McPherson's Printing Group

10 9 8 7 6 5 4 3 2 1

PEFC
PEFC/21-31-16

SAVE YOUR LIFE

& THE LIVES OF THOSE YOU LOVE

Professor Michael Kidd and Professor Leanne Rowe

Endorsed by the Royal Australian College of General Practitioners

ARENA
ALLEN&UNWIN

To our patients, who teach us every day
how to be better doctors.

CONTENTS

Acknowledgements

We wish to acknowledge the following organisations, who have developed guidelines based on research which support the recommendations in this book:

The Australian Government
The Victorian Government
Alzheimer's Australia
Arthritis Australia
Australian Drug Foundation
Australian Federation of AIDS Organisations
beyondblue
Cancer Council Australia
Diabetes Australia
Heart Foundation
Kidney Health Australia
Medibank
National Aboriginal Community Controlled Health Organisation
National Asthma Council of Australia
National Breast Cancer Centre
National Cervical Screening program
National Stroke Foundation
Nutrition Australia
Osteoporosis Australia
Prostate Cancer Foundation of Australia
Quit
The Royal Australian College of General Practitioners

We thank our colleagues from The Royal Australian College of General Practitioners, Zena Burgess, Hadia Haikal-Mukhtar, Mark Harris, Caroline Johnson, Beres Joyner, John Litt, Jane London, Ron McCoy, Chris Mitchell, Jane Smith, Teri Snowdon and Ron Tomlins for their advice on this book. We thank our great GP teacher, Professor John Murtagh. And we thank our wonderful editors, Jude McGee and Lauren Finger from Allen & Unwin.

Can you avoid death and taxes?

'In this world nothing can be said to be certain, except death and taxes.' Benjamin Franklin (1817)

Ben Franklin was right but with six easy steps, you are more likely to stay healthy, live longer and share more precious moments with the people you love. Just by improving your diet and exercising more, you could add over five years to your life and avoid many common life threatening illnesses. You could also reduce disability and do more to stop our nation's spiralling healthcare costs and free up hospital beds and waiting lists for the people who need healthcare the most. Over $1 billion of health care costs in Australia could be saved each year, if everybody exercised moderately and increased their fruit and vegetable intake by just one serve a day.

Over the past century the increase in life expectancy in this country to about 84 years of age for women and 79 for men has been achieved by advances in sanitation, immunisation and antibiotics. Unfortunately, most of the recent gains from the latest and more expensive health technology are being undermined by the impact of the current rise in obesity, inactivity and addiction rates. These conditions lead to heart disease, cancer, stroke, diabetes, respiratory disease and many other serious health problems. As a result, those affected will experience significantly more disability as they age. The life expectancy of younger generations looks like it is actually going backwards, which is extremely worrying.

Younger generations have reason to be concerned about the legacy of the over-45 age group. The high consumption of the latest expensive medical treatments for what are preventable chronic illnesses is clogging our healthcare system and will adversely affect economic growth in years to come. Already we are experiencing long delays in the public health system and private health insurance is no longer affordable for many. This crisis will worsen as the population ages, unless we start thinking seriously about prevention.

Yet most of us seem blissfully unaware of the health dangers that lie ahead. As general practitioners we often hear statements of denial like this: 'You have to die of something.' 'I'd rather die young and happy.' 'I'm better off not knowing.' 'What I don't know won't hurt me.' Australian Bureau of Statistics data reveal that while 84 per cent of the population rate their health as good or excellent, about:

- 60 per cent don't exercise enough
- 60 per cent are overweight
- 17 per cent smoke regularly
- 9 per cent consume high-risk amounts of alcohol.

As a nation we are deluding ourselves.

The fact is, our great lifestyle is killing us. Too many of us are dying prematurely or suffering the pain of chronic preventable illness.

One in two men and one in three women over 40 years of age will develop heart disease.

Approximately 820 000 Australians have diabetes with many more undiagnosed, unknowingly developing life threatening complications.

It is estimated that one in seven Australians over the age of 25 have signs of chronic kidney disease and there has been a recent 25 per cent increase in the number of people requiring dialysis.

Nearly 9000 people die of strokes in Australia each year.

One in three men and one in four women will be directly affected by cancer before the age of 75, yet many do not avail themselves of recommended screening tests for cancer.

Osteoporosis affects one in three women and one in five men over the age of 50 years.

The burden of depression and dementia is growing.

If we redirect our energy to our lifestyle and undergo screening for common health problems, much of the frailty of middle and old age can be delayed significantly.

Our book focuses on healthy living. In the first part, we provide 'six steps to staying healthy'. These actions will make the biggest difference to you, avoiding life threatening illness and adding up to five healthy years to your expected lifespan.

You may have tried to change your lifestyle before and failed. Consider these questions:

What did you learn from previous attempts to change your lifestyle?

How can you do things differently?

What concerns you at the moment and can you seek help for that?

What would have to happen for your motivation to increase?

How does your lifestyle affect your body, mood and life?

We encourage you to think about your own personalised plan and to try to set even one small goal, rather than to expect big changes all at once.

Throughout our book we refer to things we recommend you should, must or try to do, because we want to alert you to what really matters and how to prevent catastrophic illness. We want to convince you of the need to improve your health, no matter what you think your health status is at the moment. The choice is yours. You have the control to make changes.

In Part 2, we cover common preventable illnesses—heart disease, stroke, cancer, lung disease, depression, dementia, diabetes, kidney disease, osteoporosis—that cause significant disability and premature death. You will be able to identify if you are at risk of any of these illnesses, how to prevent them and how to respond to their early warning signs.

It's time for all of us to get serious about our health. Your personal health is very precious. Why wait for something to happen to your health before it becomes more important to you? Healthy living and health screening are no longer just a lifestyle choice—they are a matter of life and death. We want to help you to save your life and the lives of those you love.

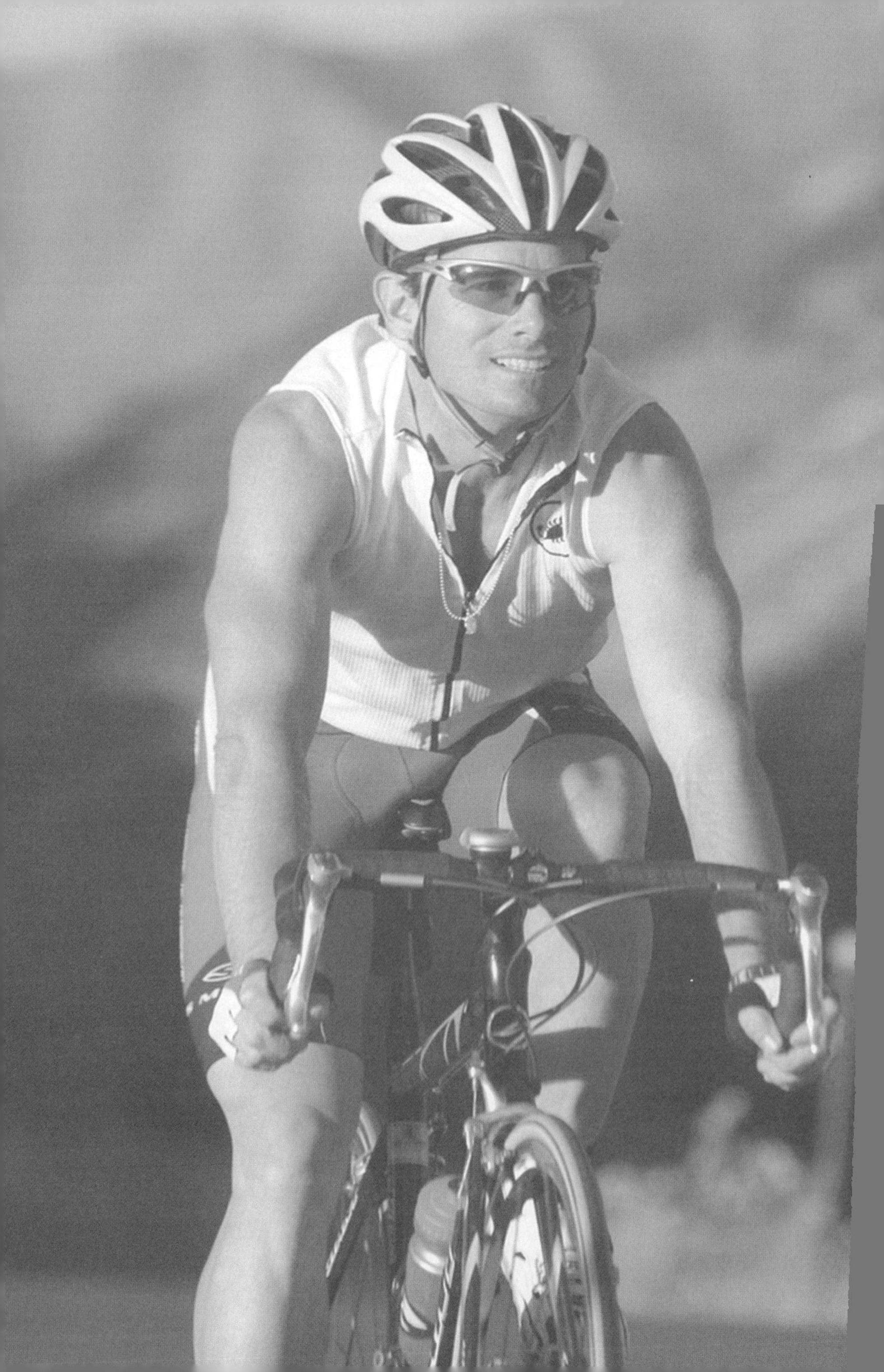

PART ONE

SIX STEPS TO STAYING HEALTHY

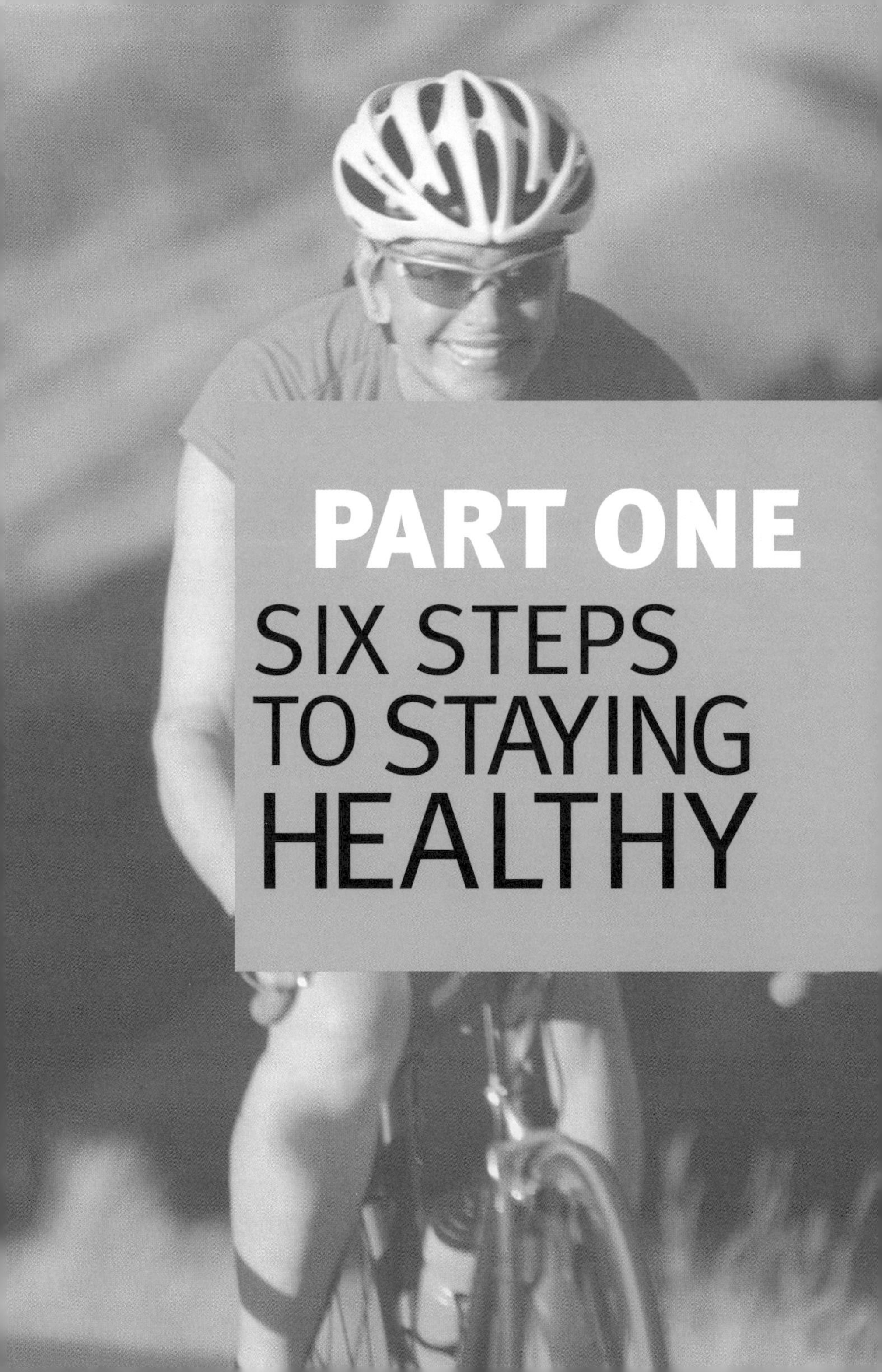

STEP 1

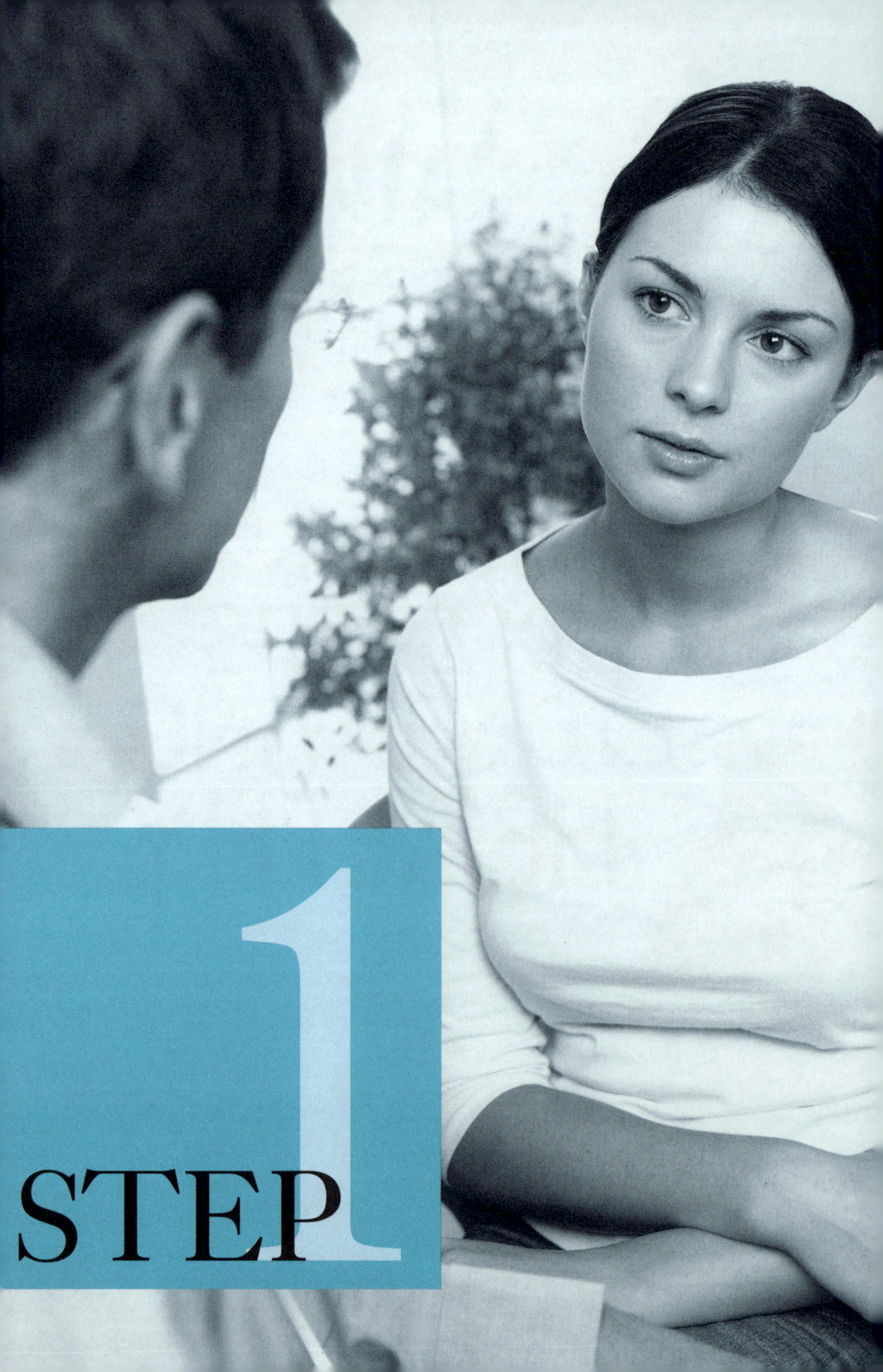

Have a check-up

Did you know that everyone over 18 should have their blood pressure measured every two years and everyone over 50, every twelve months? A preventive health check when you are healthy can be life saving, particularly for the over-45 age group. However, you may require a check-up as part of your medical care at any age, especially if you are above your healthy weight or you have a family history of illness. Your body will not automatically let you know if you have a health problem. Many preventable illnesses are silent until they are at a serious stage. A regular check-up for weight, blood pressure, cholesterol, sugar in your blood and protein in your urine, even when you feel healthy, could be life saving.

How do I choose a GP?

Your relationship with your general practitioner (GP) is crucial to your health. You should have a GP with whom you feel comfortable—someone who listens to you and shows you that they understand your concerns. A good GP is someone who:

- you can trust with confidential information
- you feel you can talk to about anything
- gives you the time you need
- uses language you can understand
- is non-judgemental about your lifestyle
- understands your culture
- answers your questions simply and honestly.

‘My husband, who was ten years older than me, passed away a year ago after being severely disabled for five years with a stroke. While I was caring for him there were times at the end of the day when I thought I couldn’t go on but I would get up the next day and it would start all over again. I recently found out my own blood pressure is up and my cholesterol is high. You really have to think about it—I haven’t been able to get myself motivated to look after myself but having a stroke like my husband would be the worst thing I could imagine.’ Margaret

Remember, this is a two-way street. Your GP may not be able to gauge what is really worrying you unless you tell her or him. The modern patient–doctor relationship is a partnership.

There are good reasons why you should try and see the same GP, or other doctors in the same medical practice, about most, if not all, your health concerns. Your detailed medical records are kept with your GP's medical practice and will include a record of the symptoms you may have experienced, as well as past diagnoses, medications prescribed, details of your social habits, your family history and your allergies. This information could be vital in helping to diagnose future health problems.

A wellness check can save your life

You don't have to feel sick to be sick. Many life threatening diseases such as heart disease, stroke, diabetes, kidney disease, cancers and osteoporosis may only be diagnosed early with simple screening tests. If you identify your risk factors for a particular disease and are diagnosed early, you are more likely to avoid serious complications and to be cured.

National expert guidelines recommend the following simple screening tests for every Australian at particular ages. Some tests may be performed by you at home and others may be performed at your general practice or your pharmacy.

From age 13 years	Skin checks for those with high risk skin by doctor For images of different skin cancers, refer to: www.sunsmart.com.au/skin_cancer/types_of_skin_cancer	Annually
From age 18 years – all the above and . . .	Waist measurement for people who appear to be overweight Waist measurement should be less than 80 centimetres for women and less than 94 centimetres for men.	Every 2 years
	Body Mass Index for people who appear to be overweight To calculate your body mass index, refer to http://home.fitness2live.com.au/body-mass-index	Every 2 years
	Blood pressure Normal blood pressure is less than 120/80	Every 2 years
	Chlamydia (urine test or genital swab) by your doctor	Annually for those at risk of sexually transmitted infections
	Mental health (including risk for depression and suicide) Refer to www.beyondblue.org.au	Every visit to your doctor as appropriate
From age 20 years – all the above and . . .	Pap smear in sexually active women	Every 2 years until age 70 years
From age 40 years – all the above and . . .	To calculate your risk of diabetes, complete the AUSRISK questionaire which may be found at: www.racgp.org.au/redbook/app2 If you have an increased risk of diabetes, your doctor will refer you for a fasting blood sugar. A glucometer reading is not an accurate measurment for the diagnosis of diabetes.	Every 3 years

From age 45 years – all the above and . . .	To determine your risk of having a heart attack or stroke you may assess your 'Absolute Cardiovascular Risk' by referring to: www.nzgg.org.nz/guidelines/0035/CVD_risk_chart.pdf If you have an increased risk of cardiovascular disease, your doctor will order more specific tests to identify and treat your risk factors to prevent a heart attack or stroke.	Every 2 years
	Fasting blood lipids or cholesterol	Every 5 years
	Osteoporosis risk assessment in women For assessment for risk factors and preventive advice, refer to: www.osteoporosis.org.au/osteo_riskfactors.php Calcium and Vitamin D supplementation is commonly required in pre and post menopausal women to prevent osteoporosis.	Annually
From age 50 years – all the above and . . .	Blood pressure more frequently	Every 12 months
	Urinary protein (tested by a 'dipstick' which is available from your pharmacy or your doctor)	Every 5 years
	Faecal occult blood Kits may be purchased at your pharmacy. The National Bowel Cancer Screening Program sends kits to people aged 50, 55 and 65 years of age only.	Every 2 years
	Prostate risk assessment in men Your doctor may refer to the guidelines at: www.racgp.org.au/policy/Prostate_screening.pdf	Risks/benefits/uncertainties of prostate screening may be discussed with your doctor.
	Osteoporosis risk assessment in men Assessment for risk factors and preventive advice	Annually
	Mammogram in women For an appointment, telephone Breastscreen on 132 050.	Every 2 years. Optional in women aged 40 to 49 and over 70.
	Vision test at your local optometrist	Every 5 years

From age 65 years – all the above and . . .	Bone mineral densitometry for osteoporosis in women by referral from your doctor	Every 2 years
	Vision and hearing tests at your local optometrist and audiologist	Annually

If you are above your healthy weight, have an unhealthy lifestyle related to poor nutrition, inactivity, smoking or excessive alcohol intake, or a medical or family history of particular diseases, or if you are of Aboriginal or Torres Strait Islander, Chinese or Indian background, some of the tests are recommended at much younger ages and at more frequent intervals.

Waist circumference and body mass index

Sixty per cent of Australians are overweight or obese.

fast facts

The total annual direct cost of obesity is approximately $21 billion in Australia.

Obesity is associated with increasing heart disease, stroke, diabetes, arthritis and some cancers. Every two years you should measure and record your waist circumference as it is used as a measure of your risk for these diseases. An abdominal circumference (on full expiration) of over 80 centimetres in women and over 94 centimetres in men increases your risk. Waist measurement is also an accurate measure of how a diet and exercise program is working on reducing your body fat. Aboriginal or Torres Strait Islander people who are over their healthy weight are recommended to have their waist circumference measured every six months.

Healthy weight is usually measured by the body mass index (BMI), which should also be calculated at least every two years. To work out your BMI follow this simple formula:

$$\frac{\text{your weight in kilograms divided by}}{\text{your height in metres} \times \text{your height in metres}}$$

As an example, Bill weighs 88 kilograms and he is 180 centimetres tall. His BMI is 27.2 (88 ÷ [1.8 × 1.8]). Generally, if you have a BMI over 25 you are at a higher risk of heart disease and diabetes. A BMI of 25 to 26.9 is associated with an eight-fold increase in type 2 diabetes compared with a BMI of less than 22. The risk increases to more than 40 times in women with a BMI over 31.

BMI	GRADE	YOUR LEVEL
below 18.5	underweight	
18.5 to 24.9	normal weight	
25 to 29.9	overweight	
above 30	obese	

Sometimes BMI may be misleading and can be confusing. For fit people with muscular bodies or those embarking on an exercise program to lose weight, an *increasing* BMI should not be discouraging as it may indicate increasing muscle bulk, which is positive. On the other hand, heart and stroke risk may increase as BMI *decreases* with muscle wasting and increasing body fat in older, inactive people.

What if your results are outside the normal range?

If your results are outside the normal range, try to set your own personal goal for weight loss by reducing the energy or kilojoule content of your diet and increasing your exercise. Many people lose weight by simply reducing their consumption of high-fat and high-sugar junk foods. The obesity epidemic has now become so serious that more aggressive treatments may be required for some people, including very low-kilojoule diet drinks, medication and laparoscopic gastric banding. (Refer to Steps 3, 4 and 5 of this book for information about healthy nutrition, exercise and ways to help you with your kilojoule balance.)

Blood pressure

About 3.7 million Australians aged over 25 years have high blood pressure and in most cases the cause is unknown. Raised blood pressure is usually silent and rarely causes headaches or other symptoms. Unfortunately, this means many people do not know they have high blood pressure so they fail to take adequate action to treat raised blood pressure and prevent its serious complications. Yet your doctor can quickly assess your blood pressure using a sphygmomanometer.

There are two blood pressure readings: the systolic pressure, which peaks when the heart pumps; and the diastolic pressure, which falls when the heart relaxes. Normal systolic blood pressure is less than 120 and normal diastolic blood pressure is less than 80. Your blood pressure is affected by body position, breathing, stress, exercise and sleep. The higher your blood pressure, the higher the risk of

TAKE AWAY MESSAGE

If a woman reduces her waist circumference to below 80 centimetres and a man below 94 centimetres, the risk of heart attack, stroke and diabetes is significantly reduced. Losing a few centimetres in waist circumference and keeping your BMI below 25 can literally add years to your life.

complications. Your risk escalates if high blood pressure is associated with high blood cholesterol, smoking or diabetes.

If you have no known health problems, you should have your blood pressure checked at least every two years before the age of 50 and then every twelve months thereafter, as raised blood pressure seriously increases the risk of heart attack, heart failure, stroke and kidney damage.

People of Aboriginal and Torres Strait Islander, South Asian or Maori and Pacific Islander backgrounds are at increased risk and should have their blood pressure checked annually from age 15.

HOW HIGH IS YOUR BLOOD PRESSURE?

Systolic (mmHg)	Diastolic (mmHg)	Grade	Your level
less than 120	less than 80	normal	
120–139	80–89	borderline	
140–159	90–99	mild to high	
160–179	100–109	moderate to high	
180 or more	110 or more	severe high	

What if your results are outside the normal range?

If your blood pressure is more than 120 over 80 on several occasions you may need to make some changes to your diet and lifestyle, including:

- reducing your weight
- improving your diet
- reducing salt intake
- increasing potassium intake
- cutting back on alcohol consumption
- giving up smoking.

Although the cause of high blood pressure that is unresponsive to lifestyle changes is largely related to family history or unknown, there are a number of illnesses that need to be excluded such as kidney and thyroid disease. If your blood pressure is still too high after making lifestyle changes, your GP will commence regular medication to prevent complications. Medication controls rather than cures the level of blood pressure and it usually needs to be taken for life.

It is important to remember that some herbal medicines such as liquorice root, ginseng and black cohosh may *increase* blood pressure.

Cholesterol

Cholesterol is a type of fat that is part of all animal cells. It is also produced in your liver. When there is too much cholesterol in the blood, fatty plaques build up in the walls of your arteries. A sudden heart attack or stroke may be the first signs that your arteries are clogged in this way.

TAKE AWAY MESSAGE

- The complications of high blood pressure are totally preventable.
- If your blood pressure is more than 120/80 on several occasions, you have high blood pressure and require immediate lifestyle changes.
- If your blood pressure does not respond to lifestyle changes medication must be commenced to prevent heart attack, stroke and kidney damage.
- The good news is that high blood pressure often responds well to simple lifestyle changes or prescription medications.

The main causes of high blood cholesterol are eating too much fat, especially saturated fat from animal sources such as full cream dairy products and meat, and being overweight. While some foods such as egg yolk, caviar, prawns, calamari and octopus contain high levels of cholesterol, these foods have less impact on blood cholesterol than saturated fat from animal sources.

A blood test for cholesterol can be ordered by your GP. The sample is taken after at least ten hours of fasting. You may consume water only, and must abstain from alcohol during this time. The blood test results are not one simple number; there are four components of the blood test results, broken down as follows:

- HDL (high density lipoprotein)—the good cholesterol; the more HDL, the better.
- LDL (low density lipoprotein)—the bad cholesterol; the less LDL, the better.
- Triglyceride—the less triglyceride, the better.

- Total cholesterol—the total of HDL, LDL and triglyceride levels. This component is not meaningful on its own but it is usually high when LDL is high.

Triglycerides are an important energy source for the body. This type of blood fat normally rises after a meal and drops as it is used by the body. High blood triglycerides are usually due to obesity and high fat, sugar and alcohol intake, and are also associated with heart disease and stroke.

Healthy men and women should start having their cholesterol measured every five years from the age of 45 or earlier, and every one or two years if there is a family history of heart disease or other risk factors such as smoking, obesity, diabetes and high blood pressure. Aboriginal and Torres Strait Islander peoples should have their cholesterol measured every year from age 18.

The normal result for total cholesterol is less than 5.5 mmol/litre; for HDL, more than 1 mmol/litre; for LDL, less than 2.5 mmol/litre; and for triglyceride, less than 2.0 mmol/litre.

What if your results are outside the normal range?

IS YOUR LEVEL TOO HIGH?	
Ideal level	**Your level**
Total cholesterol level (desirable, less than 5.5 mmol/l)	
HDL cholesterol level (desirable, more than 1 mmol/l)	
LDL cholesterol level (desirable, less than 2.5 mmol/l)	
Triglyceride level (desirable, less than 2 mmol/l)	

If your total cholesterol is high *only* because your HDL (the good cholesterol) is high, no action is required. Your level of LDL cholesterol is a better indicator of risk of heart attack and stroke than total cholesterol. If your total cholesterol is high because your LDL or your triglyceride levels are high, you will need to make changes to reduce the level of saturated fat in your diet and have your levels rechecked three months later. Unfortunately, sometimes high blood cholesterol levels are genetic and inbuilt, and do not respond to lifestyle changes.

Your GP may prescribe you a cholesterol-lowering medication in the following situations:

- Your total cholesterol is over 6.5 and your HDL cholesterol is less than 1.
- Your total cholesterol is over 5.5 and you have diabetes.

- Your cholesterol is over 5 and you have a strong genetic predisposition to heart disease.
- Your total cholesterol is over 7.5 or your triglyceride level is over 4 and you are a man aged 35 to 75 or a postmenopausal woman.
- Your cholesterol is over 9 or your triglyceride level is over 8 at any age.

You can also be prescribed these medications regardless of your cholesterol level if you are in a very high-risk category, such as if you:

- have active heart disease, stroke or arterial disease
- have diabetes associated with microscopic protein in your urine
- are an Aboriginal and Torres Strait Islander person with diabetes
- have diabetes and are in the over-60 age group
- have a family history of heart disease (where at least one close family member developed heart disease before age 45 or two close family members developed the disease before 55).

If you require medication, most commonly your GP will recommend a drug called a 'statin'—HMG-CoA reductase inhibitor—to reduce the risk of heart

TAKE AWAY MESSAGE

- Over 6.5 million Australians aged 25 and over have high levels of cholesterol.
- High blood cholesterol is a silent killer in otherwise fit healthy people—by reducing your cholesterol you can prevent heart disease, stroke, and even dementia.
- Guidelines recommend cholesterol lowering medications regardless of cholesterol levels with some medical conditions or family histories.

disease and stroke. Your blood levels of cholesterol should be monitored every six to twelve months.

If your high blood triglyceride levels are not responding to reducing weight or intake of fat, sugar and alcohol in your diet, you will also need to take a medication to help reduce your triglyceride levels. This is a different medication to the statins.

Unfortunately, about one in three people tend to discontinue cholesterol and triglyceride lowering medication, usually because they remain unconvinced about the need to take regular medication when they feel healthy. However, the benefits of lowering blood fats are proven.

Sometimes other causes of high cholesterol need to be ruled out such as thyroid problems, kidney disease, liver disease and certain medications.

> 'I was tired all the time and thought it was due to my recent weight gain. Then I went to the optometrist because my eyesight seemed to be deteriorating and I thought I needed new glasses. My optometrist picked up changes in my eyes and this means I have had the diabetes for a while, without realising it. I am now more energetic with the tablets for lowering the high sugar in my blood and I am working on my weight. My sisters have also been screened for diabetes.' Kai

Fasting sugar (blood glucose level)

Normal sugar (glucose) levels in the blood are important for energy. The blood glucose level rises after you have eaten any carbohydrate (remember, sugar is a simple carbohydrate). The blood glucose level then falls as this carbohydrate is absorbed into the cells of the body through the action of insulin, a hormone produced by the pancreas. Type 2 diabetes occurs when your cells become resistant to the action of insulin, causing your blood glucose levels to remain high.

Desktop glucometers (tests done on blood obtained by a pinprick test on the finger tip and measured in a small portable machine) and urine tests are not sensitive enough to rule out diabetes; a fasting blood test from a pathology laboratory is required.

Your GP will calculate your risk of diabetes and will recommend a blood test for glucose every three years if you are 40 years of age and over. You should start being tested from the age of 40 if you have other risk factors, such as obesity (a BMI greater than 30), or a close relative with type 2 diabetes, a history of diabetes during pregnancy or high blood pressure. Some groups of people, such as Indigenous Australians, Pacific Islanders or those from the Indian subcontinent or China, should be screened every year from 35 years. If you have borderline levels of blood sugar, high blood pressure or polycystic ovarian disease, are above your healthy weight or have had a stroke or heart attack you will require screening every year.

What if your results are outside the normal range?

If your blood test is outside the normal range you may require an oral glucose test which is a series of blood tests taken before and after a big glucose drink. The oral glucose test monitors your body's response to glucose over time. Depending on the level of your result, your doctor may advise a range of treatments, from simple lifestyle changes to medication.

IS YOUR FASTING BLOOD GLUCOSE LEVEL TOO HIGH?	
Blood glucose levels	**Your level**
Less than 5.5 mmol/litre: diabetes unlikely	
5.5 to 6.9 mmol/litre after fasting or 5.5 to 11.0 mmol/litre on a randomly tested blood sample: borderline (an oral glucose test will be done to exclude diabetes)	
7.0 mmol/litre or more after fasting or 11.1 mmol/litre or more on a randomly tested blood sample: diabetes likely	

TAKE AWAY MESSAGE

- Type 2 diabetes is often silent but symptoms can include frequency of urine, blurred vision or fatigue.
- Early diagnosis is extremely important to prevent life threatening complications.
- A simple fasting blood glucose test is recommended every three years from the age of 55 years, or from the age of 40 years if you are at a higher risk or above your healthy weight.
- Borderline raised blood glucose is often treated simply with healthy diet and exercise.
- If your BMI is less than 25 and you exercise regularly, your risk of developing diabetes is significantly less.

Urine protein test

Your urine can be a window to the internal workings of your body. Urinating frequently may sometimes indicate diabetes or infection. Difficulty starting urination in men sometimes relates to an enlarged prostate.

With a simple dipstick test in your GP's office, microscopic urine can provide a lot more information. There is no protein in normal urine. Tiny amounts of blood or protein can indicate serious illness. Blood in the urine is always significant and should be checked to exclude causes such as infection, cancer or kidney stones. Protein in the urine may be a sign of kidney disease.

To help guard against the harms of kidney disease, everyone over 50 years should have their blood pressure measured every twelve months and their urine tested for protein every five years so problems can be identified and treated early. If you have high blood pressure or a family history of kidney disease, your GP will order a urinary microalbumin test and a blood test called a glomerular filtration rate. These tests provide an accurate measure of the extent of any kidney damage that may have already occurred.

What if your results are outside the normal range?

The most common causes of kidney damage are high blood pressure, diabetes and kidney disease such as nephritis (inflammation of the kidneys) or scarring of the kidneys. Treatment of high blood pressure, high cholesterol, weight reduction and quitting smoking will prevent and treat many causes of kidney disease. For more information, refer to Chapter 8 on kidney disease.

Other tests

You can refer to Part 2 of this book for more information about the following tests:

- prostate screening (pages 109–10)
- mammogram (pages 114–15)
- bowel cancer screening (page 118)
- skin check (pages 121–22)
- pap smear (page 125)
- osteoporosis risk assessment and bone densiometry (page 171)
- visual and hearing impairment testing (page 176).

Keeping track

Your GP will be able to provide you with a list of your 'numbers' (such as blood pressure, cholesterol and

TAKE AWAY MESSAGE

- If you are over 50 years, it is recommended you have your urine tested for protein every five years to check for kidney disease.
- Microscopic traces of blood, protein or glucose in the urine are sometimes the only signs of kidney disease.

BMI) compared with normal values. It's a good idea to ask your GP for a photocopy of your pathology results and other measurements and to file them in your own personal health record at home. Your own record will help jog your memory when your next tests are due.

You may find it helpful to photocopy the following page and take it to your next check-up with your GP. Complete the sections you can and ask your GP to complete the rest. The following chapters describe your dietary and exercise requirements and the screening tests in detail. See the table on the following page.

PERSONAL HOME HEALTH RECORD			
Screening tests that your GP may recommend (normal values in brackets)	Date of test	Result	Date next due
Waist measurement (less than 80 cm in women, 94 in men)			
Body mass index (20–25)			
Blood pressure (less than 120/80)			
LDL cholesterol (less than 2.5 mmol/litre)			
Fasting blood glucose (less than 5.5 mmol/litre)			
Protein, blood, glucose in your urine			
Pap smear			
Mammogram			
Skin check for changing skin lesions			
Faecal occult blood test			
Prostate check			
Osteoporosis risk assessment and bone densitometry test			
Visual and hearing impairment testing			

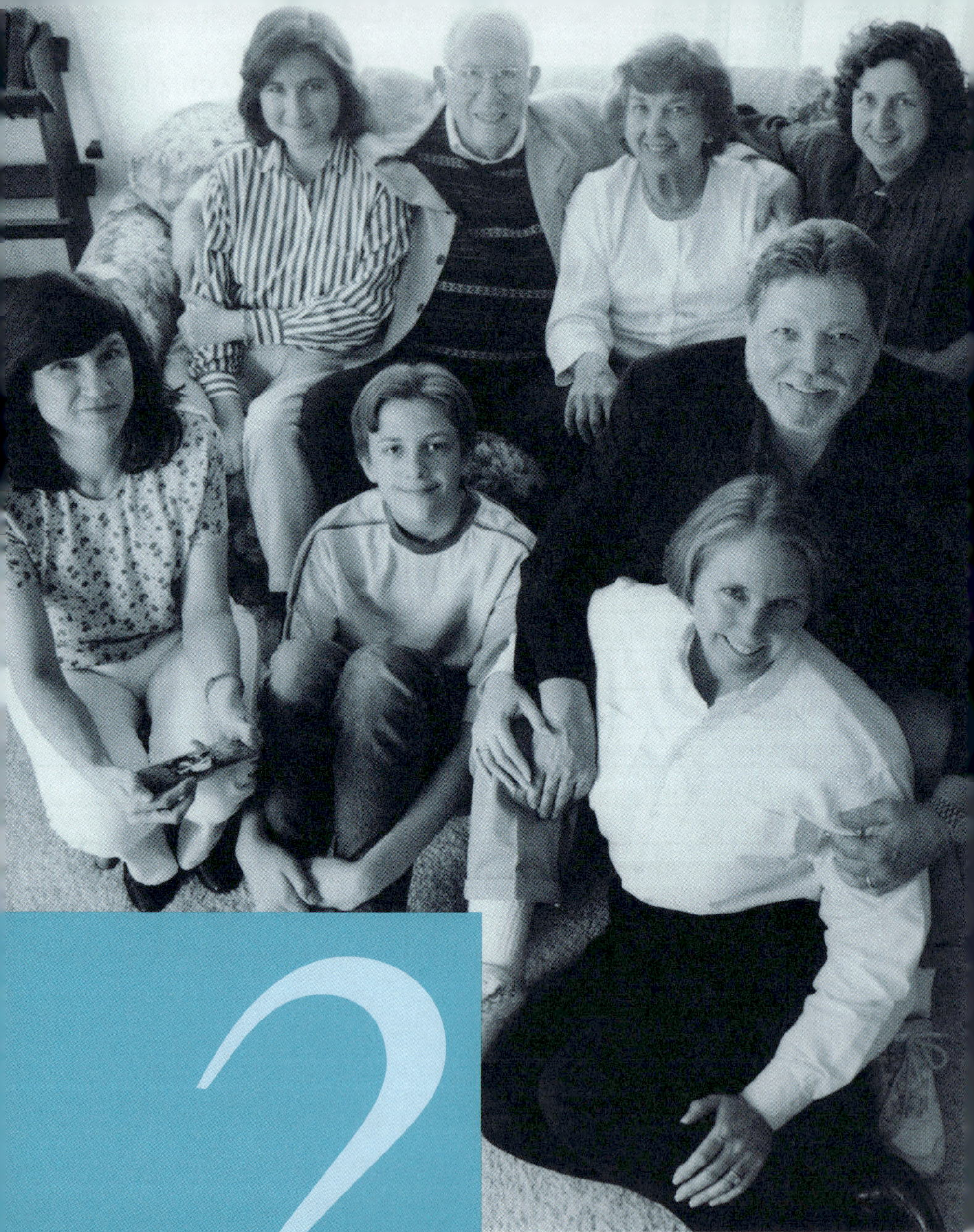

STEP 2

Know your family history

You will find it easier to develop your own personal health plan if you know your family history. Many common health problems run in families and have a genetic basis. Your family history determines when you require screening for particular illnesses, what areas of your health you and your GP need to focus on and when and how often you need to screen for illness. Having a comfortable relationship with the same GP will encourage you to seek healthcare when you need it—early.

As examples, a healthy 45-year-old, slim, athletic woman, whose mother died of a heart attack suddenly at the same age, may be at the same high risk but requires a different approach from an overweight 45-year-old man who smokes and has two sisters with diabetes. Although she is very fit, the slim athletic woman might have high cholesterol and high blood pressure, and she could suffer the same fate as her mother. The man who smokes on the other hand has a very high risk of undiagnosed diabetes. His smoking may have already contributed to arterial disease affecting his heart, brain, kidney, limbs and eyes. These complications may only become apparent at the end stage of the disease, when it may be too late to help. In both cases, simple tests ordered by a GP will help prevent years of disability or premature death.

While other specialists may focus on their particular area of expertise, your GP will look at you as a whole person and provide advice on your total health. In the

‘I have always taken my health for granted—my grandparents on both sides lived well into their eighties and most of them smoked. But now I've found out my younger sister has bowel polyps and high cholesterol. My older sister found out she has osteoporosis after fracturing her ankle after a fall. They did the right thing and had things checked out, so I thought I should see my GP to work out what I should do.’ Jessica

first case, the athletic woman should have blood pressure and cholesterol checks every two years. She should pay attention to reducing the saturated fat in her diet and keeping her cholesterol low. In the second case, the man with a strong family history of diabetes should have an early screening test for glucose and any borderline result followed up closely. He would be very wise to stop smoking, exercise more and adopt a low-fat, high-carbohydrate (low glycaemic index) diet to protect his health in the future.

Everyone's needs are different. Your GP will help you develop a plan that suits you.

Start by recording your own medical history and then list anything you know about your immediate family members. Discuss what you are doing with family members and ask them to disclose their medical history to you. Contact the registry of births, deaths and marriages to explore details on death certificates of family members who have passed away. You could use the list below as a guide.
In the 'other' column, note conditions like:

- alcoholism or drug dependency
- blood disorders
- high blood pressure
- high cholesterol
- epilepsy
- eye disorders, such as blindness, cataracts
- kidney disease
- liver disease
- musculoskeletal disorders, such as arthritis
- psychiatric disorders such as depression or schizophrenia
- lung disorders such as asthma.
- dementia
- osteoporosis.

Try to confirm your family history with health records, and note the age when any diagnosis was made and how seriously it impacted upon the health of your family member or their age at death.

With this information, ask your GP to formulate your family 'tree', to record your full family history and to determine what screening tests you need and when you need them.

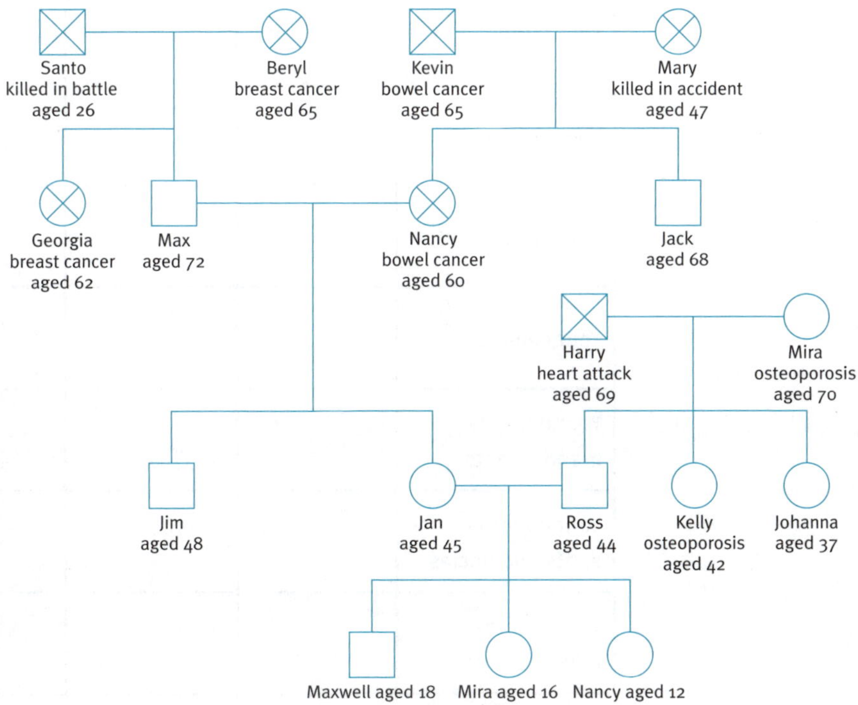

Jan has a family history of breast cancer and bowel cancer.
Ross has a family history of heart disease and osteoporosis.

Family member	Names	Alive or deceased	Current age or age at death
You			
Your children			
Your mother			
Your father			
Your brothers			
Your sisters			
Your cousins			
Your maternal grandparents			
Your maternal aunts and uncles			
Your paternal grandparents			
Your paternal aunts and uncles			

-leart disease or stroke (age of onset)	Type 2 Diabetes (age of onset)	Type of cancer (age of onset)	Any other conditions (age of onset)

As already discussed, screening tests are routinely recommended to measure your weight, blood pressure, cholesterol, glucose and urine protein at particular ages. If you have a family history of diabetes, heart disease, stroke, kidney disease or certain cancers, you require earlier screening, depending on the age at which your relative acquired the disorder. There are other disorders such as psychiatric illness, drug dependency, epilepsy, blindness, arthritis and asthma which also run in families and contribute significantly to disability. If you have a family history of any of these conditions, inform your GP, especially at the first signs of any worrying symptoms. For example, if you have a family history of asthma and find it difficult to exercise due to breathlessness, you may have exercise-induced asthma, which may require treatment. If you have a family history of rheumatoid arthritis and you start to experience joint pains in your fingers, you will benefit greatly from having an early diagnosis and appropriate treatment of the condition. If you have persistent headache and a close family history of ruptures of blood vessels in the brain, you may require imaging of your brain to exclude an aneurysm, which is an abnormal blood vessel with a tendency to rupture.

There are a number of genetic tests now available which are appropriate for certain conditions where an individual is considered to be at risk. These conditions include breast cancer, cystic fibrosis, Down syndrome, haemachromatosis, colon cancer, thalassaemia and fragile X syndrome. Genetic centres offer good genetic counselling, predictive genetic testing, medical advice and psychological support for people concerned about inherited disorders. People who have three or more close relatives with a particular cancer, for example, may wish to know what their inherited risks are, to discuss the advantages and disadvantages of genetic testing and, if tested positive, determine the frequency of screening for the disorder.

Unfortunately a small number of people will request expensive and unnecessary medical investigations to temporarily soothe their fear of a rare fatal disease: 'Just give me all the tests.' 'I'd like a back X-ray just to be sure.' 'I'd rather see a specialist to rule out everything serious.' We are not advocating over-investigating. An example of medical technology gone mad is regular, total body CT scan screening, which is an enormous waste of time, money and anxiety, and which exposes people to high doses of radiation. False positive results from unnecessary screening can lead to even more invasive and expensive tests. We strongly recommend against unnecessary screening. If you are concerned, speak to your general practitioner. If you don't have a GP, it is time to find one who you can trust and who can assist you to balance the risks and benefits of any investigation or treatment.

TAKE AWAY MESSAGE

Consult your GP to develop a total personal health plan for screening for common, preventable illnesses, based on your medical history and your family history.

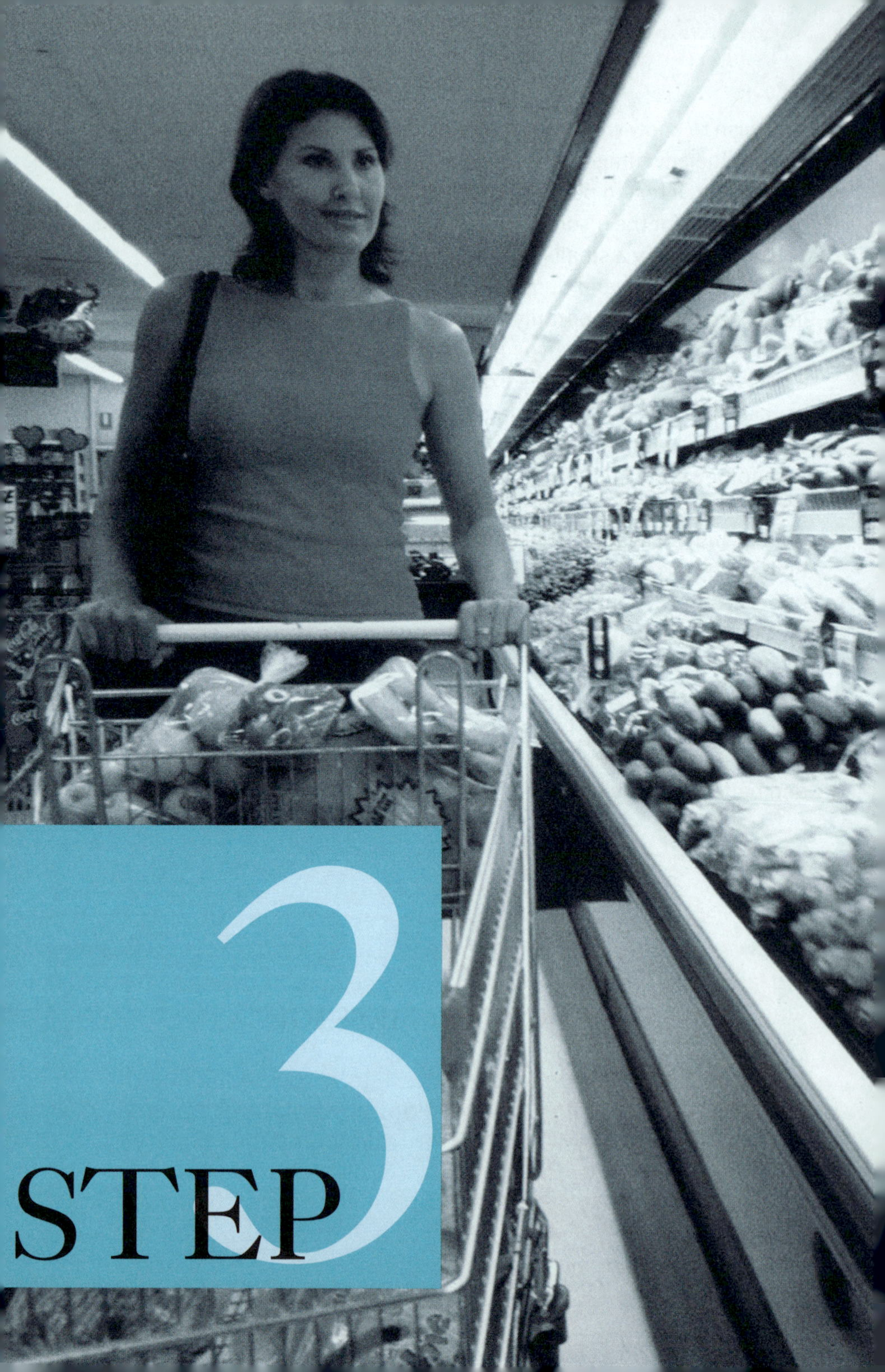

STEP 3

Improve your diet

Good nutrition is the basis of a long and healthy life. We recommend a diet that is high in low glycaemic index carbohydrates, and low in saturated and trans fats. This diet will give you the energy you need to increase your exercise, help you lose weight permanently and help protect your health against heart disease, stroke, diabetes, some cancers and osteoporosis.

Being above your healthy weight is associated with serious consequences and obesity requires aggressive management with medical treatments, if healthy nutrition and exercise fail.

Sixty per cent of Australians are overweight or obese. Illnesses related to poor diet, such as heart disease, diabetes and osteoporosis, are on the increase. There is an enormous amount of media and public interest in unproven, quick-fix fad diets. If you visit your local bookstore, you will see there is no shortage of best-selling books on diets that don't work. Many diets are difficult to maintain in the long term and leave you feeling exhausted, unwell, hungry or flatulent. In this situation your weight tends to yo-yo, leaving you discouraged and depressed.

Choice of food can be confusing. Even the choice of spread to use on your bread can be complicated. But there is no mystery surrounding Australia's epidemic of obesity: we are simply eating more kilojoule-rich foods and exercising less. Food is

'Last weekend I went away and ate what everyone else ate but I put on two kilos. When I felt fat and depressed I binged on things I know I shouldn't eat. I need the motivation to start a diet again just to lose a few kilos. I know what to do, I just can't do it.' Trinh

energy and we need to eat only as much as we can burn. If you want to lose weight, energy taken in should be less than energy expended.

Let's get back to the basics of a good, common sense diet. A good diet:

- provides you with enough energy and can therefore be sustained in the long term
- maintains your healthy weight
- keeps your arteries unclogged (prevents heart disease)
- stabilises your blood glucose (prevents diabetes)
- builds your bones (prevents osteoporosis).

About one third of the dollars spent on food in Australia is spent on restaurant and takeaway foods. We are what we eat, but often we are not aware of what we are eating.

What is a balanced diet?

Healthy nutrition means eating a variety of foods at regular times throughout the day to maintain your energy levels without causing large rises in your blood glucose levels. Healthy meals are based on high-fibre carbohydrate foods such as wholegrain breads and cereals (oats, barley, psyllium, porridge, untoasted muesli), legumes (dried beans, lentils, chickpeas), raw vegetables and salads (leafy green vegetables, carrots, tomatoes, and cruciferous vegetables like broccoli, cabbage, brussels sprouts, bok choy and other Asian greens) and fruit (citrus fruits are particularly high in antioxidants). Dietary guidelines recommend a daily intake of two to four serves of fruit and four to eight serves of vegetables. Foods containing calcium and iron are encouraged while fat, particularly saturated fat (meat, full-cream milk and other diary products), sugar and salt are discouraged. Healthy snacks include fruit, wholegrain bread, raw vegetables, a small quantity of nuts and seeds and low-fat milk or low-fat, plain yoghurt. Two or more serves of oily fish (salmon, sardines, herrings, mackerel, tuna and trout) per week are recommended. Water and green tea are the best drinks.

How does food work?

To understand this, you must first understand the basic components of food and their kilojoule or energy content.

Kilojoules

When you regularly eat more energy than your body needs, the excess is stored as fat. If you reduce your activity levels, as happens as you grow older, but continue to eat the same amount of food, you will gain weight.

Kilojoule refers to how much energy a food contains and how much energy is burned up during exercise. For example, an apple contains 330 kilojoules and a blueberry muffin contains 1120 kilojoules. Prior to metric measures we used calorie. (One calorie has the same energy value as 4.186 kilojoules.) Just one kilogram of body fat contains the equivalent of 37 000 kilojoules. Healthy weight loss therefore does not occur quickly. Fast weight loss with fad diets is often related to a temporary loss of fluid and loss of muscle. To lose one kilogram of body fat in a week, you would need to burn an additional 37 000 kilojoules, or around 5000 kilojoules a day.

Carbohydrates are most readily converted to energy and are the body's preferred energy source. Fats

(37 kilojoules per gram) and alcohol (29 kilojoules per gram) are by far the most energy dense foods, so they should be consumed only in moderation as they promote weight gain most easily. Fatty, sugary, processed and fast foods are a readily available quick-fix for fatigue, but in the long term, junk food contributes to chronic tiredness and ill health.

Fat

Fat has a high energy value of 37 kilojoules per gram and therefore promotes weight gain. Total dietary fat intake must be cut if you want to lose weight. Sometimes this can be achieved by simple methods, such as changing to a low-fat cooking method of baking like steaming. The type of fat you eat is also important. For instance, saturated fat in meat and full-cream dairy products clogs arteries as it increases blood fats. The risk of heart disease and stroke can be reduced by decreasing the amount of saturated fat in your diet.

Polyunsaturated, mono-unsaturated and saturated fatty acids may be broken down differently in the body. Some fats, like polyunsaturated fats (especially omega-3 fatty acids from fish oils), may be used up more easily from fat stores during exercise than saturated fats from other animal sources and are less fattening. Although saturated fats are more fattening, all fried foods, even those cooked with poly- or mono-unsaturated fats, promote weight gain.

Protein

Protein has an energy value of 17 kilojoules per gram. Protein is required for the growth and repair of the body but many protein foods, such as meat, contain fat. Although helpful in controlling appetite, high-protein diets based on meat and dairy products (which are high in saturated fat) can increase your risk of heart disease in the long term. The best protein foods to choose are those that are low in fat, like:

- dried peas, beans and lentils
- fish and seafood, lean meat and poultry without the skin
- low-fat or skim-milk dairy foods, such as milk, yoghurt and cheeses such as cottage or ricotta.

An adequate intake of protein without increasing the risk of heart disease may be consumed through 65 to 100 grams of lean meat or chicken or 80 to 120 grams of fish, three to four times a week.

Carbohydrates

Carbohydrates have an energy value of about 16 kilojoules per gram. Carbohydrates are broken down by the body into sugars or glucose. The type of carbohydrate you eat is important as carbohydrates with a low glycaemic index stabilise your blood glucose and your level of hunger and energy because they are absorbed more slowly. The glycaemic index tells us if a carbohydrate food will raise blood glucose levels a little, moderately or dramatically. The glycaemic load of a food relates to the glycaemic index and the quantity that would normally be consumed in a serve. Low glycaemic foods such as wholegrain bread, fruit and vegetables are recommended to prevent and treat diabetes. Noodles, brown rice and pasta are other examples of low glycaemic index foods.

Poor energy levels and sugar cravings are aggravated by high glycaemic index carbohydrate foods because your blood glucose tends to rise and fall quickly. Diets of high glycaemic index carbohydrate foods (such as high-sugar drinks, confectionery, cakes, biscuits and pastries) tend to be more fattening than lower glycaemic index foods. High glycaemic index foods also increase the risk of heart disease by increasing the level of triglyceride in the blood. In general, the sweeter the taste of food and the lower the fibre content, the higher the glycaemic index.

Do you need to change your diet?

If you have a waist circumference over 80 centimetres (women) or 94 centimetres (men) or a BMI over 25, you must lose weight to maintain your health. Even if your measurements are normal, think about your family history and if your risks for any illnesses are increased. For example, if you have a family history of heart disease, diabetes or osteoporosis, you may need to make adjustments to prevent future health problems, even if your cholesterol, blood glucose and bone densitometry tests are normal now.

Obesity has now reached epidemic proportions in many developed countries and has very serious consequences. Your choice of food significantly influences your short-term and long-term health. Obesity treatment requires an aggressive approach, with options ranging from low-kilojoule diets, use of a food diary to identify emotional eating, low-calorie drinks and diet pills, to laparoscopic gastric banding.

The first five kilograms seem to be the hardest to lose and the easiest to regain for most people. The most common reason fad diets fail is that they can't be maintained in the long term due to side effects or because rapid weight gain is related to *temporary* loss of fluid or muscle loss from the diet, resulting in dehydrated skin and unattractive, flabby muscles.

Another reason fad diets fail is that they don't recognise the underlying problem of an emotional appetite. By identifying your emotional appetite and how you respond by eating, you will become more aware when you are eating for comfort rather than nutrition.

Weight-loss diets have been shown to be much more effective when a food diary is used to monitor food intake. If you are unable to recall your food intake over a week or even a few days, just think of a typical day. Identify your hungry times of the day and circle your unnecessary kilojoule-rich foods. Include the amounts and type of food, drinks (milk, alcohol, soft drink), sugar, salt, spreads, takeaway food and food eaten between meals while on the run, cooking or cleaning up. Include all the 'extras', such as that odd chip left over on a child's plate. For each entry, include alcohol and smoking, identify your mood and pinpoint how you are feeling. For example:

- Have you just eaten a packet of chocolate biscuits after being insulted by your neighbour?
- Do you get home from work exhausted and order takeaway and flop into your TV chair with a glass of wine?
- Do you rush out of the house without eating breakfast and then purchase a muffin for morning tea?
- Do you feel guilty when you eat the wrong foods and then eat more?
- Do you shop when you are tired and hungry and bring home chips, chocolate and soft drink?

Stand back and look at the way you use food to satisfy your 'emotional appetite'.

Food diary (note kilojoule level per serve of food consumed from food label on a jar, bottle or can)				
Day/time	Food or drink, including alcohol	Quantity and kilojoule content	Place where eaten	Mood at the time/ other events

Look at your entries and see if you can you make small changes, such as getting up 15 minutes earlier in the morning, going for a walk or doing relaxation exercises to release tension, or precooking your dinner for exhausting days at work or home.

After reviewing your record of a 'typical day', set a few goals for improving the next week, such as:

- changing to a healthier morning tea
- increasing fruit intake
- cutting unnecessary treats
- reducing the size of your dinner meal
- eating less fatty, fried food
- cutting down red meat and full-cream dairy products
- introducing a wholegrain breakfast.
- drinking water instead of soft drink or alcohol.

From the food diary you will be able to identify times of the day when you are susceptible to poor eating and drinking habits and how this relates to your mood. Think about other ways you can respond to negative emotions rather than eating. Plan to replace high-kilojoule, high glycaemic index foods and drinks with low-kilojoule, low glycaemic options. Reduce fats, particularly saturated fat. Eat more fibre- and antioxidant-rich foods. Decrease your non-hungry eating and eat more slowly. Plan your individual diary for the following week.

People who lose weight successfully set goals and rewards, weigh themselves regularly, eat healthy food consistently with no days off and exercise opportunistically and regularly.

WHAT IS A HEALTHY SNACK?

Avoid eating between meals if you can. Try drinking water first. If you crave food in between meals try a small serve of the following:

- **raw vegetables like carrot and celery**
- **fruit**
- **low-fat plain yoghurt or low-fat milk**
- **unsalted almonds**
- **wholegrain bread.**

Which diet should you choose?

The low-fat (particularly low saturated fat), high-carbohydrate (particularly high-fibre, low glycaemic index carbohydrates) diets are the most effective for keeping weight, cholesterol, blood pressure and risk of diabetes down. High-protein diets (such as the Zone diet, Protein Power diet and the CSIRO diet) assist some people to lose weight and reduce triglyceride levels, but may have adverse effects in others by reducing kidney function and increasing the risk of bowel cancer (if the protein is based on red meat and processed meat). Some of these problems may be overcome if fish and chicken are substituted as the source of protein and the fibre content of the diet is increased. If you have metabolic syndrome (obesity, high cholesterol, high glucose, high blood pressure), you may require more restriction of carbohydrate and fat. In this case a diet proportionally higher in protein may be helpful. The Atkins diet is a low-carbohydrate diet that is difficult to maintain and can lead to raised LDL cholesterol, constipation and vitamin and mineral deficiencies. The South Beach diet is like the Atkins diet but replaces saturated fat with unsaturated fat and has not been studied in the long term.

IDENTIFY ACTIVITIES YOU CAN DO INSTEAD OF EMOTIONAL EATING
For instance, talking over a problem with a friend, walking, relaxation exercises, listening to music, gardening, knitting, playing sport.

There is no magic bullet for losing weight. It takes willpower. The overall goal of any diet or treatment should be to establish a pattern of healthy living you can maintain. Healthy nutrition and exercise are the basis of a long and healthy life; however, there are a number of treatments available that may help you shift stubborn kilograms and give you the motivation to keep persevering. For example, very low-calorie meal replacements can be an effective option for weight loss. They are balanced nutrient mixes that reduce portion size and energy intake and are usually used to replace one or two meals a day.

Diet pills have side effects, are expensive and are not recommended without lifestyle changes or for long-term use.

Weight-reducing medications increase the metabolism of the body and some have an antidepressant effect. Some inhibit the digestive enzymes that break down fat and may be better tolerated than other diet pills. However, as dietary fat is not absorbed, it sometimes passes through the bowel undigested as diarrhoea. Others contain a molecule that creates feelings of fullness, blocks weight gain and blocks out the receptors in the brain that transmit pleasure from eating. Side effects of these prescription tablets may include hyperactivity, palpitations, high blood pressure, dry mouth and headache. However, these side effects are immediately reversible when the medication is stopped. If you are considering taking weight-reducing medication, discuss this with your general practitioner.

Surgery can be life saving for some people with obesity. Laparoscopic adjustable gastric banding (LAGB) is increasingly recommended for people who are seriously obese (with a BMI over 40 or BMI over 35 with medical conditions). LAGB surgery has been found to be effective in reducing obesity in the long term, and can lead to improvements in people with diabetes, high cholesterol, sleep apnoea and high blood pressure. Unfortunately, some people maintain the attitude that surgery for obesity is cosmetic and should be confined to privately insured patients. This attitude discriminates against people who are obese.

Food labels and how to read them

Take time to eat fresh food and try to avoid packaged processed food. If you purchase anything in a jar or plastic package, read the food label carefully for kilojoule, fat and sugar content. Apart from the fact that many people cannot read the tiny font of food labels, it is difficult to assess the nutritional value of food from the food label alone. Sometimes foods are low in fat but high in sugar and low in fibre. As trans fats are not saturated they are not listed separately on food labels, so the unsaturated fat profile can look deceptively good.

Some food labels can be misleading.

- '90% fat free' is actually still high in fat.
- Cheese is often labelled as reduced fat if it is 25 per cent fat.
- 'Lite' or 'light' may relate to taste or salt, not fat content.
- 'Cholesterol-free' products may include coconut and palm oil, which are high in unhealthy saturated fat.
- 'Toasted' usually means fattier rather than healthier—toasted muesli has twice the fat of non toasted muesli.

To avoid confusion, look for the Heart Foundation tick, which is applied to foods that are low in saturated fat. According to the Heart Foundation, 'low fat' means less than 3 per cent for solids and less than 2 per cent for liquids.

The 'GI' symbol indicates the glycaemic index rating of packaged food products in supermarkets. GI ranks food products based on the speed at which they break down from carbohydrate to sugar in the bloodstream but the GI symbol will only appear on food products that meet certain nutrient criteria for that food category. High and intermediate GI soft drinks, cordials, syrups, confectionery and sugars, jams, honey and other carbohydrate-containing spreads may be excluded from labelling.

Other beneficial food components

Phyto-estrogens are found in soybeans, lentils, beans, chickpeas, wholegrain cereals, seeds, apples, carrots, garlic, linseed, alfalfa and clover sprouts. There are positive effects of phyto-estrogens associated with better heart function but no conclusive evidence on them reducing menopausal symptoms, cancer or osteoporosis.

Recent studies on coffee have shown that moderate intake has no adverse effects on health. Dark chocolate, however, has clear cardiac benefits, blood pressure reduction and decreased inflammation and may be even more beneficial to health than tea and red wine with higher antioxidant levels.

Antioxidants in citrus fruits, berries, vegetables, lettuce, broccoli and cauliflower counteract free radicals. Free radicals are damaging molecules caused by pollution, smoking, sunlight and X-rays, and can promote ageing, cancer, heart disease, Alzheimer's disease, arthritis and blindness.

There is no evidence that vitamin supplements are necessary for prevention or treatment of heart disease or other chronic disease in well-nourished healthy people. A well-balanced diet is preferable.

Anaemia

Iron deficiency anaemia can occur in vegetarians, people who have diets low in meat or premenopausal women. Anaemia is a common cause of fatigue and difficulties with thinking and concentrating. Iron supplements are sometimes necessary for vegetarians or in women, particularly those with heavy menstrual bleeding. However, dietary adjustments can also be effective in correcting anaemia without increasing red meat.

Good sources of iron include tofu, legumes (lentils, dried peas), wholegrain cereals (in particular, iron-fortified breakfast cereals), green leafy vegetables such as spinach, nuts such as cashews, fruits such as dried apricots, eggs and seeds such as sunflower.

Vitamin C has been shown to enhance the absorption of the non-haem iron found in plant foods by up to two to three times if taken at the same time. So to improve your iron intake, combine iron-rich plant foods with foods that are rich in vitamin C, such as citrus fruits, fruit juice, berries, tomatoes, capsicum, broccoli and cabbage.

Tannic acid is a substance that can interfere with the absorption of non-haem iron, reducing it by as much as half. To ensure an adequate iron intake, avoid drinking tea, coffee and cola drinks (which all contain tannic acid) at meal times.

TAKE AWAY MESSAGE

- Weight loss and long term good-health are best achieved by a diet low in fat and high in carbohydrates (low glycaemic index), and increasing exercise.
- Try to identify your emotional eating habits, reduce non-hungry eating and eat more slowly.
- People who lose weight successfully set goals and rewards, weigh themselves regularly, eat healthy food consistently with no days off and exercise opportunistically and regularly.
- Meal replacements, diet pills and gastric band surgery are effective in treating obesity, but should only be considered in combination with lifestyle changes.

STEP 4

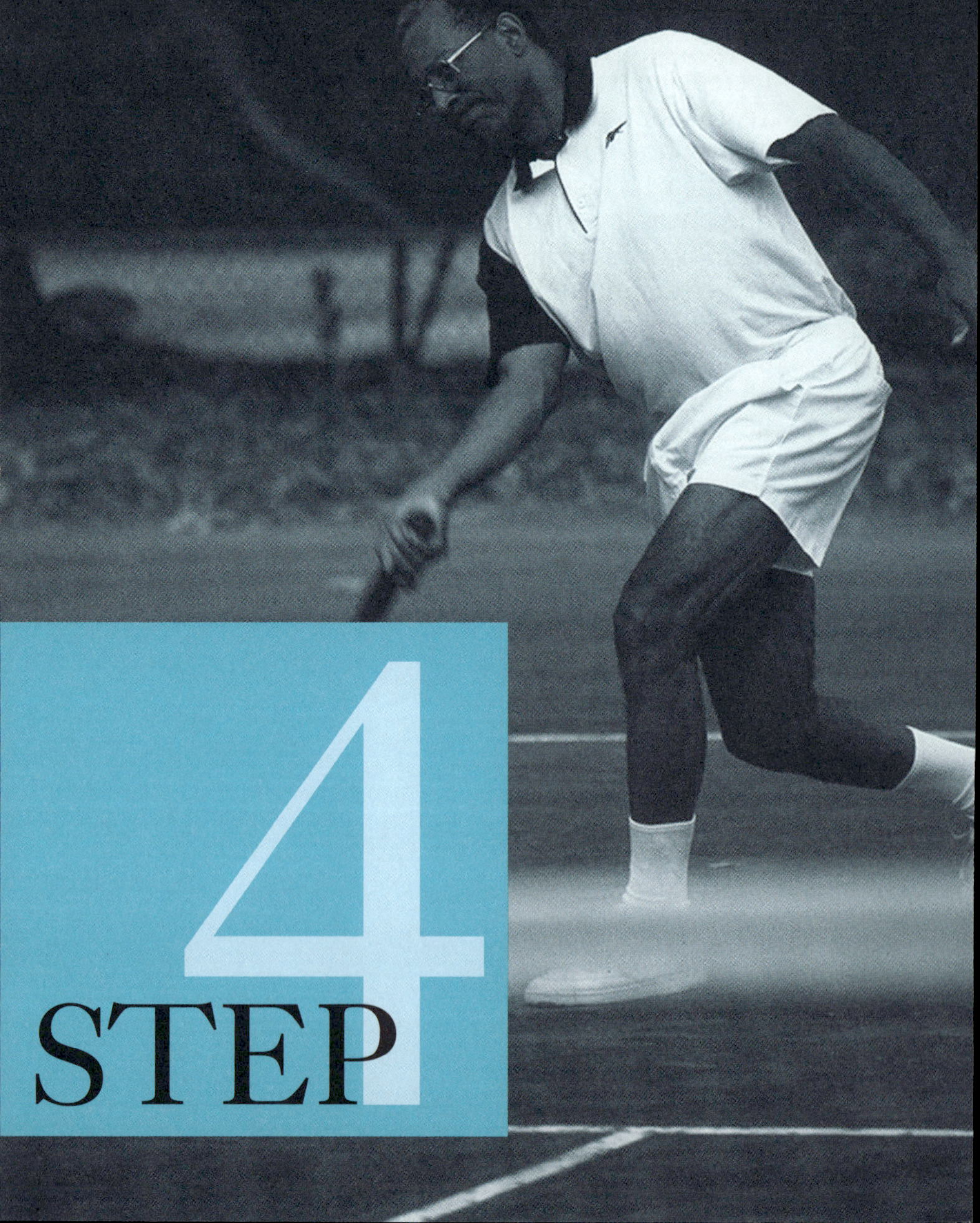

Exercise more

fast facts

It is estimated that physical inactivity alone costs $1.5 billion each year.

Sixty per cent of Australians are inactive. Exercise is essential for good health, relaxation and healthy body weight. If you engage in moderate exercise daily, you will add, on average, up to four years to your life. The benefits are greater for more vigorous exercise.

Regular exercise is essential for health and full of benefits. It can:

- keep your weight down as body fat increases when energy absorbed from food is more than the energy expended by exercise
- keep your blood pressure down
- raise the good cholesterol in your blood (HDL) and lowers the bad cholesterol (LDL) and triglycerides
- help prevent type 2 diabetes, stroke and heart disease
- reduce stress, depression and other mental illness
- strengthen your bones
- delay the onset of dementia
- help reduce the risk of cancer and better outcomes after cancer diagnosis, particularly bowel cancer and breast cancer.

‘I know I should exercise more but there’s no way I can fit it in. I get home from work late and flop in front of the TV with a beer. I had the best intentions and then wasted a gym membership. I’m too tired to exercise.’ Josh

What kind of exercise is good for you?

It does not matter what kind of exercise you do, the most important thing is that you enjoy it and that your heart rate increases while you are doing it. Weight bearing exercise will also strengthen your bones and includes walking, running, aerobic exercises, dancing and lifting weights. Other exercise to consider includes swimming, cycling, pilates and yoga.

Exercise is being 'engineered' out of our lives through labour-saving technology. If you are having trouble fitting exercise into your daily routine, make simple changes like using the stairs, parking further away from your workplace or shopping centre, and walking to school with your kids. Don't make your exercise plan too complicated or let it defeat you. An expensive gym membership is not necessary.

How much exercise should I do?

Exercise is classified into moderate and vigorous. Moderate exercise will cause a slight, but noticeable, increase in breathing and heart rate and may cause light sweating in some people. To work out your ideal heart rate during moderate exercise, calculate your maximum heart rate in beats per minute by subtracting your age from 220. If you have cardiovascular disease or other serious illness, you should discuss how to exercise safely with your GP. Use the chart opposite to find out your maximal heart rate.

To calculate your ideal heart rate during moderate exercise take 60 to 70 per cent of your maximum heart rate in beats per minute. This is the rate you need to aim to attain for a minimum of 30 minutes five times a week. This amount of exercise may help maintain your weight rather than lose weight. If you wish to lose weight you simply need to exercise for longer and stimulate your heart rate more every day.

Age	Maximum heart rate (220 minus your age)	Moderate exercise (60 to 70 per cent of your maximum heart rate)
30	190	114–133
40	180	108–126
50	170	102–119
60	160	96–112
70	150	90–105

While moderate exercise is recommended for a health benefit, more vigorous exercise may confer additional heart health if carried out for a minimum of 30 minutes three to four times a week. Vigorous exercise is activity that leaves you huffing and puffing so that it's difficult to talk in full sentences between breaths. During vigorous exercise aim for a heart rate that is 70 to 85 per cent of your maximum heart rate. Work out your rates and write them in the worksheet for reference.

MINIMUM REQUIREMENT OF EXERCISE FOR HEALTHY PEOPLE	YOUR LEVEL
Your maximum heart rate (220 minus your age)	
During moderate exercise, your heart rate will be at least ______ (60 to 70 per cent of your maximum heart rate)	
During vigorous exercise, your heart rate will be at least ______ (70 to 85 per cent of your maximum heart rate)	

Remember, though, the duration of exercise is more important than intensity. Whatever exercise you choose, measure your heart rate to monitor your progress.

How can I build exercise into my day?

Lack of time for exercise is the most common reason given for sedentary lifestyle. Family and work commitments often take priority. But you owe it to yourself, your family, your friends and your work colleagues to take time to exercise. You will stay healthier, feel more energetic, take less sick leave and live longer. Think about ways to build exercise into every day of your life. Try some of these simple steps:

- get up earlier and exercise
- go for a walk at lunch time
- use the stairs rather than the escalator or elevator
- go for a walk after work instead of flopping in front of the TV
- enlist the support of a walking companion—a family member, friend or a dog will help you keep to the routine
- walk when you do your errands
- go exploring to a different park, walking track or around a shopping market or museum
- meet friends for a walk, rather than a coffee
- take up a social sport—anything—self defence, tennis, golf, yoga
- try gardening
- hire a treadmill if you get home after dark
- make an appointment with yourself each day to do some exercise and don't cancel.

How can I stick to an exercise plan?

Sticking to an exercise plan is more about your mindset than anything else. Don't make it too complicated. Place this list of questions on your fridge at home and work and answer them honestly.

1. Why is there always something more important to do than exercise?
2. What are the benefits of changing my attitude to exercise?
3. What are my lifestyle stresses?
4. What are the good things about living this way? What are the less good things?
5. What's stopping me from exercising?
6. What are the consequences of not doing anything for my health?

Remember:

- Be convinced of the benefits of exercise—it can add years to your life whatever your health status.
- Persevere through the initial discomfort—with regular exercise you will find it easier.
- Keep it simple—do any exercise you enjoy.
- Measure your heart rate and aim to increase it—set realistic goals.
- If time is a problem, try three lots of ten minutes of exercise each day—get up ten minutes earlier and go for a walk, take time out again at lunch time and again before your evening meal.
- Reward yourself with something like a low kilojoule treat or an MP3 player or some new running shoes.
- Use a pedometer and aim to walk over 10 000 steps each day.
- Try to set a goal like beating your pedometer reading or training for a charity walk or marathon.

- Treat any medical problems restricting your exercise promptly—don't break your exercise habit.

Common causes of exercise intolerance

Asthma should not restrict exercise. (Chapter 4 covers the treatment of asthma, including exercise-induced asthma.) Asthma should be adequately treated to allow normal exercise. Talk to your GP.

Joint pain can make exercise extremely hard work. About 30 per cent of people aged 40 and over have back pain that interferes with exercise. Regular walking and activity are good ways to prevent and also treat back problems.

Osteoarthritis, the most common form of arthritis, usually found in the knees, neck, lower back, hip and fingers, is a very common reason why people over 40 do not exercise. While movement sometimes temporarily aggravates the pain of arthritis, regular exercise improves chronic pain in the long term. Hydrotherapy is a non-weight bearing form of exercise that can be particularly helpful. Glucosamine sulphate and chondroitin, available from your chemist, may help take the edge off the pain of osteoarthritis.

Consult your GP before you suddenly embark on a vigorous exercise program or if you have a condition that restricts your ability to exercise. If you experience any temporary chest pain during exertion, stop immediately and see your GP as soon as possible. If chest pain is not relieved by rest, go immediately to your closest accident and emergency centre by ambulance.

TAKE AWAY MESSAGE

Moderate physical activity like brisk walking, swimming or cycling is recommended on most, preferably all, days of the week, for about 30 minutes a day. The duration of exercise is more important than the intensity. Most of all do something you enjoy and will maintain. Take time to relax.

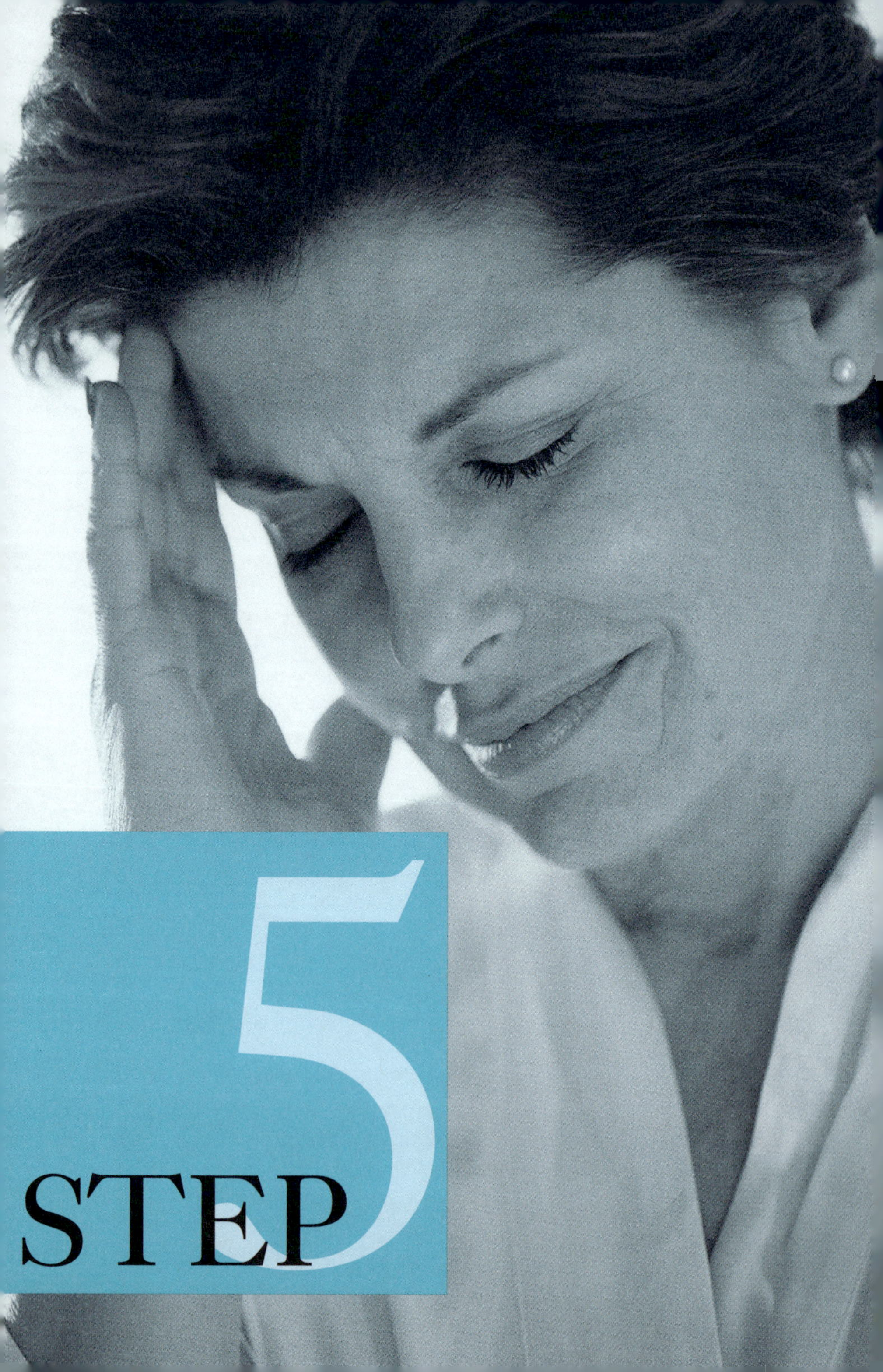

STEP 5

Reduce your risky behaviours

Some bad habits like smoking, alcohol or other drugs are temporary quick fixes for stress. In the short and the long term, bad habits can create major health problems and even more stress.

Reduce unhealthy stress

Sometimes stress causes a natural 'fight and flight' bodily reaction where your level of adrenalin increases and your awareness of your surroundings is heightened. This reaction allows you to take the necessary steps to protect yourself from harm or future stress. More often, your body's reaction to stress is a bad habit and damaging to your health and your immune system. It may be helpful to think about your 'stress bucket'. List the sources of your stress (the things that turn on the taps and overfill your stress bucket). Now think about what helps you release stress and the steps you have to take to keep the bucket from overflowing.

The sources of your stress may include poor nutrition, smoking, heavy alcohol intake and concerns about your health, along with concerns about your family, other relationships and work. If you are smoking, drinking alcohol excessively or using illicit drugs to try to release your stress, understand that this drug use also adds to your levels of tension. You are more likely to release stress if you talk to someone about your concerns, seek help and make changes to

'I thought if someone told me I had to quit smoking for a medical reason, I would just do it. The doctors told me to stop smoking and taking the pill when I had the stroke. Well I've stopped the pill but I just can't stop smoking.' Emma

In tap: What makes your stress bucket overfull or overflow?

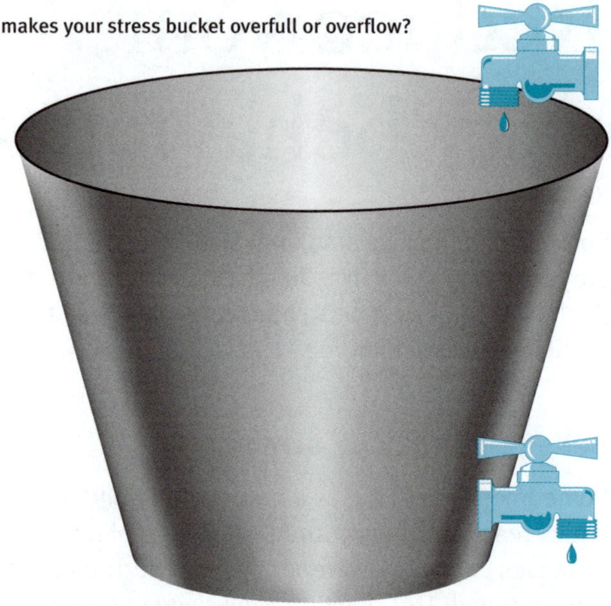

Out tap: What helps you release the water pressure in your stress bucket?

your lifestyle, and make time to exercise and relax. Think about how much a chronic illness or disability caused by stress or the loss of someone you love through a drug problem would add to your life stress.

The good habit of relaxation

Relaxation is extremely important for your physical and mental health and boosts your immunity. There are a number of easy strategies you can practise each day as a habit, including mindfulness, muscular relaxation, breathing retraining and visualisation.

Mindfulness

Mindfulness is a relaxed state of mind where you feel as though you are watching your thoughts as an observer. It is not a matter of stopping stressful thoughts but allowing them to flow through your mind and observe them from a distance. Sometimes the statement, 'just relax', can make things worse because your active mind finds it difficult to stop thinking and worrying. Mindfulness allows you to accept your active mind, while you step aside from the thoughts to reduce your body's over reaction.

The following techniques of muscular relaxation, breathing retraining and visualisation may help you achieve a state of mindfulness.

Muscular relaxation

Let your thoughts just flow through your mind while you tense and relax each muscle group as follows.

- Hands: Make a fist with each hand and let go and relax.
- Arms: Stretch your arms out in front of you, raise them high up over your head and stretch higher. Let your arms drop back to your side and feel them go floppy.
- Shoulders: Pull your shoulders up to your ears. Hold in tight and then relax.
- Jaw: Clench your teeth together really hard. Then let your jaw hang loose.
- Face and nose: Make lots of wrinkles on your forehead, and crinkle up your nose, then let your face go smooth.
- Stomach: Pull your stomach in. Make it touch your backbone. Get as skinny as you can, then release your stomach.
- Legs and feet: Push your feet and toes down on the floor. Let your feet and toes go loose and floppy.

Breathing retraining

This method of relaxation helps to reduce your respiratory rate. In turn, this reduces your fight and flight reaction and controls the unpleasant nervous bodily reactions to stress like sweating, flushing, shaking, over breathing or diarrhoea.

Count the number of breaths you take over one minute. Then close your eyes. Take a deep breath in through the nose and hold for ten seconds. Breathe in for the count of three seconds, and then out for three seconds.

While you repeat this for one minute, focus your attention on your breathing and counting. Keep it smooth. Expand your diaphragm on your breath in and keep your chest still. Take another deep breath in and hold for ten seconds, then breathe out for three seconds. Then open your eyes and check your resting breaths over one minute.

You will usually find your breathing rate has naturally slowed down.

Visualisation

Visualisation of past pleasant experiences is a powerful way to instant relaxation. Think of one of your favourite places, like the beach, a mountain trail, a desert oasis or a bush valley. Imagine the smells, sounds, touch and scenery. Try to feel a wonderful state of quietness and peace in this place. Feel a contentment and the warm glow. Take a deep breath in and out.

TAKE AWAY MESSAGE

Relaxation is a healthy habit. It does not matter what you do to relax, just enjoy doing it and do it regularly.

Smoking

If you are reading this chapter and you smoke, chances are you have tried to quit in the past. You know smoking is damaging your health and quitting will add years to your life, but you still can't stop. It may help to know that most people make several attempts at quitting before they succeed.

Firstly you need to know what smoking is really doing to you and be convinced of the reasons why you need to quit—now. Secondly, you will find it helpful to seek counselling and other treatments that will work.

What cigarettes do to your body

The graphic dangers of smoking are illustrated on every cigarette pack. The complications of smoking are serious and very distressing. All forms of smoking are damaging, including passive smoking, low-tar cigarettes, cigars and roll-your-own, including cannabis. There is no safe form of smoking.

Every year about 19 000 Australians die from smoking-related diseases. Smoking kills about 50 per cent of the people who are long-term smokers and causes about 40 per cent of all deaths in men and about 20 per cent of all deaths in women under 65 years. It accounts for about 300 000 admissions to hospital each year. On the other hand, it's never too late to experience the benefits of quitting smoking. The most obvious and immediate benefits are for your heart, arteries, lungs and eyes.

Smoking has been proven to cause:

- emphysema
- chronic bronchitis
- lung failure
- lung cancer.

Lung cancer is the most common cause of death from cancer in Australia. Up to nine out of ten lung cancers are caused by smoking, including passive smoking. Once diagnosed, lung cancer has a very poor prognosis and usually cannot be cured. Female deaths from lung cancer have increased seven-fold in the last 50 years.

Smoking also causes:

- other cancers, including tongue, mouth, throat, nose, nasal sinus, voice box, oesophagus, pancreas, stomach, kidney, bladder, ureter, cervix and bone marrow (myeloid leukaemia), and is linked to colorectal and liver cancer
- heart disease and heart attack—smokers are more likely to die suddenly from heart attack
- strokes
- damage to the arteries in the legs and arms which may result in pain, gangrene and the need for amputation
- aortic aneurysm (rupture of the main artery in the body)
- cataracts and other eye damage
- delayed wound healing
- much higher risks for serious complications during and after surgery
- infertility
- low bone density and hip fractures
- premature birth and low birthweight among infants of pregnant women who smoke
- periodontitis, a common dental disease, resulting in tooth decay and tooth loss.

Smokers are more likely to have:

- earlier onset of illnesses associated with diabetes, including blindness and kidney failure

- an impaired immune system
- problems with getting or maintaining an erection in men
- reduced semen volume and sperm count and more abnormal sperm compared to non- or ex-smokers
- increase in complications for women taking the contraceptive pill, including stroke and heart attack
- missed periods and more painful periods in women
- earlier menopause and more menopausal symptoms in women
- more pronounced facial wrinkling and ageing.

Smoking is also associated with severe mental illness, hearing loss and back pain. Other effects on physical appearance include staining of fingers and teeth, bad breath and a black hairy tongue.

Children who are exposed to passive smoking are more likely to die from sudden infant death syndrome and to have more infections.

Develop a plan to stop smoking

Despite the health hazards of smoking, about 3 million Australians smoke regularly because beating nicotine addiction is tough. Quitting requires a lot of support and determination. Here are a few strategies that work:

- Understand what smoking is doing to your body and that it is never too late to stop smoking to experience the benefits of quitting.
- Identify support people willing to encourage you through this difficult time, including non-smoking family members and friends.
- Set a quit date and prepare yourself for the challenge ahead.

- Ring the Quitline to talk to a supportive, independent advisor or access the website for more information.
- Avoid the triggers to smoke in the first few weeks of quitting, including friends who smoke, places that allow smoking and activities you previously associated with smoking.
- Practise saying 'No thanks. I don't smoke now'.
- Beat unpleasant cravings with simple responses like deep breathing, eating healthy food, drinking water, going for a walk, taking a bath or shower, or cleaning your teeth.
- Reward yourself with simple pleasurable things with the money you save from quitting, like a new pair of running shoes or a holiday.
- Assess your level of nicotine addiction and ask your GP for advice on nicotine replacement treatments or other medication.

Getting help to quit

How do you feel about your smoking at the moment? What are the things you like and don't like about smoking? What is motivating you to continue smoking? Are you thinking of quitting in the near future? Try to answer each question in turn to explore why you smoke and what your barriers are to quitting.

Be convinced that many of the effects of smoking may be reversible if you quit now. Do you know that some of the health benefits of quitting are immediate? Within twelve hours, the nicotine in your blood stream will have been metabolised and within twenty-four hours, your carbon monoxide levels will have dropped. After five days, your taste begins to improve and after six weeks your skin and lungs will have improved making exercise easier. Your risk of wound infection after surgery will reduce. Lung function within three months of quitting will significantly increase and after one year your extra risk of heart disease from smoking is about half, compared with people who smoke.

Ask yourself why you want to quit and what has stopped you from trying in the past. Identify what situations make you feel like smoking and how you can deal with this.

Talking about quitting helps

Most treatments fail because they are used in isolation without adequate support. It cannot be emphasised enough that talking with a supportive friend, counsellor or GP works. Talking about how you feel helps to cement the conviction in your mind to quit. It gives you confidence in your ability to succeed. It helps you make and sustain your change in attitude.

Behavioural therapy is an important first step. It encourages you to talk about the good and the bad things about smoking. It identifies your real concerns and the barriers to successful treatment and how to address them. It clears up your ambivalent feelings and helps your motivation to persevere. It challenges negative thinking and brings out your strengths to overcome your dependence.

Overcoming nicotine addiction

To grade your level of nicotine addiction, think about your level of craving, sadness, insomnia, irritability, frustration, anger, tension, difficulty concentrating, restlessness and increased appetite or weight gain after you stop smoking. Start a diary and record your feelings. If you cannot overcome negative feelings and you crave a cigarette, nicotine replacement therapy may help you.

It also helps to assess your level of nicotine dependence by the number of cigarettes you smoked on average each day and your pattern of use. Record your level in the table below.

NICOTINE DEPENDENCE	YOUR LEVEL
High dependence: more than 30 cigarettes per day, or smoking within five minutes of waking	
Moderate dependence: 21 to 30 cigarettes per day, or smoking within 30 minutes of waking	
Low to moderate: 11 to 20 cigarettes per day, or smoking within one hour of waking	
Low dependence: up to ten cigarettes per day, or not smoking within one hour of waking	

Nicotine replacement therapy

Nicotine replacement therapy often fails because inadequate doses are used. Be aware that if you smoke 20 cigarettes a day, smoke within 30 minutes of waking, or are overwhelmed by the negative feelings associated with craving, as listed above, you may require larger doses of nicotine replacement.

Sometimes the withdrawal symptoms from smoking are incorrectly attributed to side effects of nicotine replacement therapy. As a general rule if you smoke within 30 minutes of waking, try to use

4 milligrams of gum or 21/24-hour patch initially. Patch, gum, inhaler, lozenge and sublingual tablet (under the tongue) are all equally effective. Use the treatment for approximately 12 weeks in reducing doses, as directed by your GP or pharmacist. Combination treatments may be helpful if you experience withdrawal symptoms with one kind of therapy. For example, it may help to use 2 milligram gum at risky times of the day, in addition to 15 milligram 16-hour patches every day. Talk to your GP.

Prescribed medication

Your GP can prescribe certain medications in combination with behavioural therapy, if nicotine replacement therapy does not work. The oral tablets need to be taken one to two weeks before your target quit day and continued for at least seven weeks. It can be more effective than nicotine replacement therapy, but it is sometimes associated with side effects, including high blood pressure, seizures and hypersensitivity reactions. It is the preferred treatment for people who are depressed. If used in combination with nicotine replacement therapy, it requires close supervision as a likely side-effect of raised blood pressure can occur.

Other treatments, like acupuncture and hypnotherapy, do not seem to work in a significant proportion of smokers. There are a number of new treatments under evaluation, including a vaccine.

TAKE AWAY MESSAGE

One in six Australians are regular smokers, despite the graphic warnings on every cigarette pack. It is well known that smoking causes an enormous burden of illness, disability and death and that quitting greatly improves health and adds years to your life. New treatments for nicotine dependence help, but smokers require support to beat their addiction. Seek help to quit now—either via the Quitline, your pharmacist or your GP.

fast facts

Direct health costs from smoking are approximately $1.1 billion per year in Australia.

Alcohol

A lot of Australians are deluding themselves about the health benefits of alcohol. About 3000 deaths a year are directly attributable to alcohol, mainly related to liver cirrhosis, road injuries, stroke, suicide or alcohol dependence. About 70 000 Australians are admitted to hospital each year, for injury related to alcohol intake. Alcohol is the major contributing factor to violence and is responsible for a form of dementia. Statistics show that nearly 9 per cent of Australians drink at levels which are a risk to their health.

Alcohol is high in kilojoules and drinking excessively increases body weight, raises blood pressure and blood triglyceride levels. Consuming alcohol increases the risk of cancers of the mouth, pharynx, larynx, oesophagus and liver, with the risk even greater in those people who smoke. Alcohol has also been associated with colon, breast and rectal cancers.

While a small daily intake of red wine (one standard drink a day for women and two standard drinks a day for men) has been shown to reduce the risk of heart disease, stroke and dementia, if you're a non-drinker, don't start; if you're a drinker, don't start drinking more!

How much do you drink?

Think about a typical day. Ask yourself why you really need that drink at the end of the day or why you occasionally wipe yourself out with alcohol on a weekend. You may be able to identify safer forms of relaxation.

Alcohol affects different people in different ways. There is no set amount of alcohol that is safe for everybody. Use of alcohol always is a potential risk to your health and well being.

The alcohol guidelines recommend no more than an average (over one week) of two standard drinks a day (never more than four on one day), with one to two alcohol-free days each week. These drinks should be spread over several hours. Men are advised to have no more than two standard drinks in the first hour and no more than one per hour after that. Women should have no more than one standard drink per hour.

A standard drink is equivalent to 10 grams of alcohol. This means:

- light beer: 425 millilitres or a large glass
- full beer: 285 millilitres or a medium glass
- wine: 100 millilitres
- spirits: 30 millilitres
- port or sherry: 60 millilitres.

Many glasses contain more than the standard drink, so beware.

How can you cut down?

Whether you drink a little too much or have a serious drinking problem, there are a number of simple ways to cut down your alcohol intake.

- Never drink alcohol to quench your thirst and alternate between alcoholic and non-alcoholic drinks.
- Choose low-alcohol beer or dilute alcoholic drinks with mixers.
- Take smaller, slower sips and set a mental limit on your intake.
- Binge drinking is a serious health risk and drinking in shouts should be avoided for this reason.

Do you have a drinking problem?

If you feel you should cut down or if you feel defensive if someone comments on your alcohol intake, think about your level of drinking. Look for these early signs and use the simple steps above to cut down your use.

You have a drinking problem if:

- you feel agitation or other withdrawal symptoms after abstaining for a short time

- your alcohol intake is difficult to control, you abandon your usual activities because you need a drink, you are waking with a hangover or find you are spending more time trying to obtain alcohol
- you are regularly drinking early in the day.

Serious medical, psychological, relationship, legal, work and financial problems usually arise in the course of alcohol abuse.

Alcohol abuse is most obvious when people cannot fulfil their work or personal obligations due to their drinking, and alcohol is used in risky situations and continued despite the problems.

If you or someone you love has an alcohol problem, consult with your GP or local community health or drug and alcohol service to obtain information about treatment options.

Illicit drugs

Illicit drugs are a major health risk and are associated with contracting HIV, hepatitis B and C and mental illness. People who use illicit drugs are at risk of becoming malnourished and overdosing. Illicit drugs include cannabis, inhalants, heroin, ecstasy, LSD, amphetamines and cocaine.

Cannabis or marijuana is very harmful. It is associated with loss of energy and motivation, impaired concentration, depression, anxiety and psychosis. Lung disease and cancer are also more common as roll your own cigarettes have more tar than commercial cigarettes.

Solvents or inhalants such as volatile substances like paint thinner and gasoline, and aerosol sprays may be associated with long-term damage to the

TAKE AWAY MESSAGE

A small amount of alcohol may have health benefits, but many people are drinking at high-risk levels. Injuries related to alcohol result from violence, accidents, falls, having unprotected sex and alcohol poisoning. Long-term harm from alcohol includes diseases such as cancer, diabetes and damage to liver and brain cells. Most of the short- and long-term adverse effects of heavy alcohol are reversible. For all these reasons, it's important to cut down your level of alcohol intake. The benefits of drinking less alcohol will be immediate. You will feel sharper and more energetic.

nervous system, kidneys, liver and heart and sudden death.

Heroin is a highly addictive drug that slows the bodily functions. Withdrawal symptoms are severe and overdose is common.

LSD (lysergic acid diethylamide) is a hallucinogenic and addictive drug that causes paranoia, confusion and acute panic. Long-term effects include intense nightmares and mental illness.

Amphetamines such as speed, ice or crystal stimulate the nervous system and in high doses may cause seizures, strokes, paranoia, hallucinations and aggressive behaviour.

Ecstasy causes hallucinations, thirst and overheating. Death may occur with excessive fluid intake. It impairs memory and may cause permanent brain damage.

GHB is a liquid anaesthetic which can cause loss of coordination, nausea, dizziness, breathing problems, loss of consciousness and death, especially when combined with alcohol and other drugs.

Cocaine causes heightened awareness, anxiety and paranoia. In higher doses it may result in aggression and hallucinations. Like other stimulant drugs, overdose can cause death due to seizures, heart attacks, brain haemorrhage, kidney failure or stroke.

Intravenous drug use and sharing injection equipment is related to the transmission of blood-borne viruses such as HIV and hepatitis C and B. Safe injecting practices can help protect against infection. Needle and syringe exchange programs are run by health departments in each state.

Unfortunately illicit drug use is often related to underlying mental illness and addiction. If you can't stop your drug use, professional help is necessary to reduce the harm of ongoing drug abuse. Consult your GP or community health service or drug and alcohol service for further assistance and appropriate referral.

Steps to reduce your drug use

There is no safe level of illicit drug use. The aim of drug treatment is to reduce your use and the harm associated with it. Try to buy less, set limits, put your smoking and other gear away, and plan for drug-free days. Ask for support from someone who will encourage you and help you deal with conflict, stress, boredom, guilt, anxiety and grief in other ways.

It may help to sort out your feelings and identify why you have a problem with a certain drug in the first place. What do you like about using the drug? What would be good about reducing your drug use? What don't you like about your drug use? What would make it hard to cut down?

Cravings after stopping drug use are normal—you may feel like a hungry feral cat and the cravings will continue if you keep feeding your habit. Think about what may help to distract you from your cravings. Try drinking more water, exercising, resting, baths, massage, reading, sport, art, music, making plans for the future, camping, bushwalking, gardening, dancing or yoga. Reduce other stimulants such as tea, coffee, cola drinks and sugar. If you mix tobacco with cannabis, nicotine replacement therapy may help.

Reassure yourself that the common withdrawal symptoms of drug addiction will pass and try to ride through them. Withdrawal usually lasts from four days to two weeks and can be unpleasant: disturbed sleep, bad dreams, mood swings, headaches and tiredness, irritability, nausea, hot and cold flushes, lethargy and tremors are common.

Most importantly, don't give up if you relapse and find you start using again. Ask yourself what you will do differently in the future. Self-help is not easy. Ask for support from a family member, friend, GP and community health centre or drug and alcohol service.

TAKE AWAY MESSAGE

Illicit drugs are more harmful than you think. Quite apart from the content and dose being unknown, illicit drugs cause serious side-effects, dependency and are associated with mental illness. Drug treatment often requires support, counselling and replacement medication to overcome dependency and addiction.

Unsafe sex

The good news is that safe sex is great for your health. The health advice website of the National Health Service in the United Kingdom recently reported that sex relieves stress, soothes pain, cures insomnia, makes your hair shine, vanishes wrinkles, protects against prostate cancer, slows the ageing process, stimulates the body's immune system, reduces cholesterol levels and lowers the risk of heart disease!

Perhaps some of these claims may be a little far fetched, but what we can be sure about are the dangers of unsafe sex. Unsafe sex can lead to serious infections such as HIV, syphilis, hepatitis, herpes, gonorrhoea, chlamydia and warts. Some of these

fast facts

Sexually transmissible infections, such as HIV, syphilis, gonorrhoea and chlamydia, are on the increase in Australia. Chlamydia is one of the most common sexually transmissible infections (STIs) in Australia, especially among young people.

infections can be life threatening, others can cause serious long-term illness. Some sexually transmitted infections may have few or no symptoms until the disease becomes serious and advanced.

Safe sex is any sexual activity that prevents body fluids, such as semen, vaginal fluids or blood, from entering the bloodstream of another person. The use of condoms and water-based lubricant can prevent fluids entering the body during vaginal or anal sex. Anal or vaginal sex without condoms remains the most common high risk sexual activity for transmitting HIV.

fast facts

It is very worrying that about 1000 new cases of HIV are diagnosed every year in Australia. HIV remains one of the greatest health risks to men who have sex with other men.

There are many reasons why people have unsafe sex. It may be related to the use of alcohol or other drugs. It may occur when people have sex with a new partner or are beginning a new relationship. It is important that you know what is safe and what is not. If in doubt, talk to your general practitioner or consult a reputable website.

The most common notifiable sexually transmitted infection in Australia is chlamydia. Chlamdyia is a serious cause of infertility and pelvic pain in women. Chlamydia may cause a urethral discharge in men or a vaginal discharge in women. However, it can also cause no symptoms at all. All women and men at risk of sexually transmissible infections should be screened for chlamydia every year. Those infected should be screened again after six to twelve months because of the high risk of reinfection. The sexual partners of people with chlamydia should also be tested and treated.

People at high risk of chlamydia infection should be screened every twelve months. This includes men who have anal sex with men; all sexually active teenagers, especially females; and all people with a pattern of inconsistent or no condom use, or with a recent change of their sexual partner. Screening for chlamydia involves a urine test, or a vaginal swab. The mouth and anus may also be swabbed if appropriate.

It is important that you are able to talk to your treating doctor openly and frankly about your sexual health. If you have unsafe sex and are at risk of a sexually transmitted infection, or if you think you may have a sexually transmitted infection, consult your general practitioner or local sexual health centre.

TAKE AWAY MESSAGE

- Safe sex is good for your health.
- Unsafe sex is extremely risky behaviour.

Avoid accidents

fast facts

- The most common accidents in Australia are: car accidents, drowning, falls, poisoning, burns, and industrial and farming accidents.
- The most common risk factor for accidents is alcohol.
- Major trauma is the leading cause of death in Australians aged under 44 years.

Accidents are an avoidable cause of serious disability and death. How do you reduce your risk of becoming an accident statistic?

The most common cause of accident deaths and disability is transport-related accidents, such as car and motorbike accidents and pedestrian accidents. Up to 30 per cent of fatal transport accidents are related to driver fatigue. The warning signs of fatigue include:

- yawning
- eyes feeling heavy
- difficulty concentrating
- hunger
- unintentional variations in speed.

Strong coffee or a power nap are the only measures that work to combat driver fatigue.

Try to avoid common distractions while driving such as smoking, adjusting audio equipment, use of mobile phones, reading or writing, or personal grooming.

RISK QUIZ

DO YOU DO ANY OF THE FOLLOWING?		
Do you always wear a seat belt when travelling by car?	Yes	No
Do you always drive at a safe speed and within the speed limit?	Yes	No
Do you avoid driving when you are fatigued?	Yes	No
Do you avoid driving under the influence of alcohol or other drugs?	Yes	No
Do you avoid using your mobile telephone while driving?	Yes	No
Do you take particular care each time you cross a road?	Yes	No
Do you follow all the occupational health and safety guidelines for your work?	Yes	No
Do you think twice before you climb a ladder to ensure that all is safe?	Yes	No
Do you always take care when swimming in the ocean or a river?	Yes	No
Do you have fire fighting equipment (fire extinguisher, fire blanket) at your home and work?	Yes	No
If you are aged between 50 and 64, do you have your vision checked every five years?	Yes	No
If you are aged 65 years or over, do you have your hearing and vision checked every year?	Yes	No

If you answered 'No' to any of the above then you may be placing yourself and other people at increased risk of serious injury or death due to an accident.

You should choose a safe speed for the road conditions at the time. Speed limits are the maximum safe travel speeds recommended for any road. When the weather is bad or when the traffic is heavy or when driving after dark, you should consider travelling at a lower speed.

The sudden and unexpected nature of injury from major trauma can make dealing with it especially difficult, for both the injured person and their family and friends. Support and counselling are often beneficial. This can be a key role for your general practitioner.

TAKE AWAY MESSAGE

- Always wear a seat belt.
- Don't drink and drive.
- Avoid distractions when driving.
- Have a power nap or strong coffee if feeling fatigued.

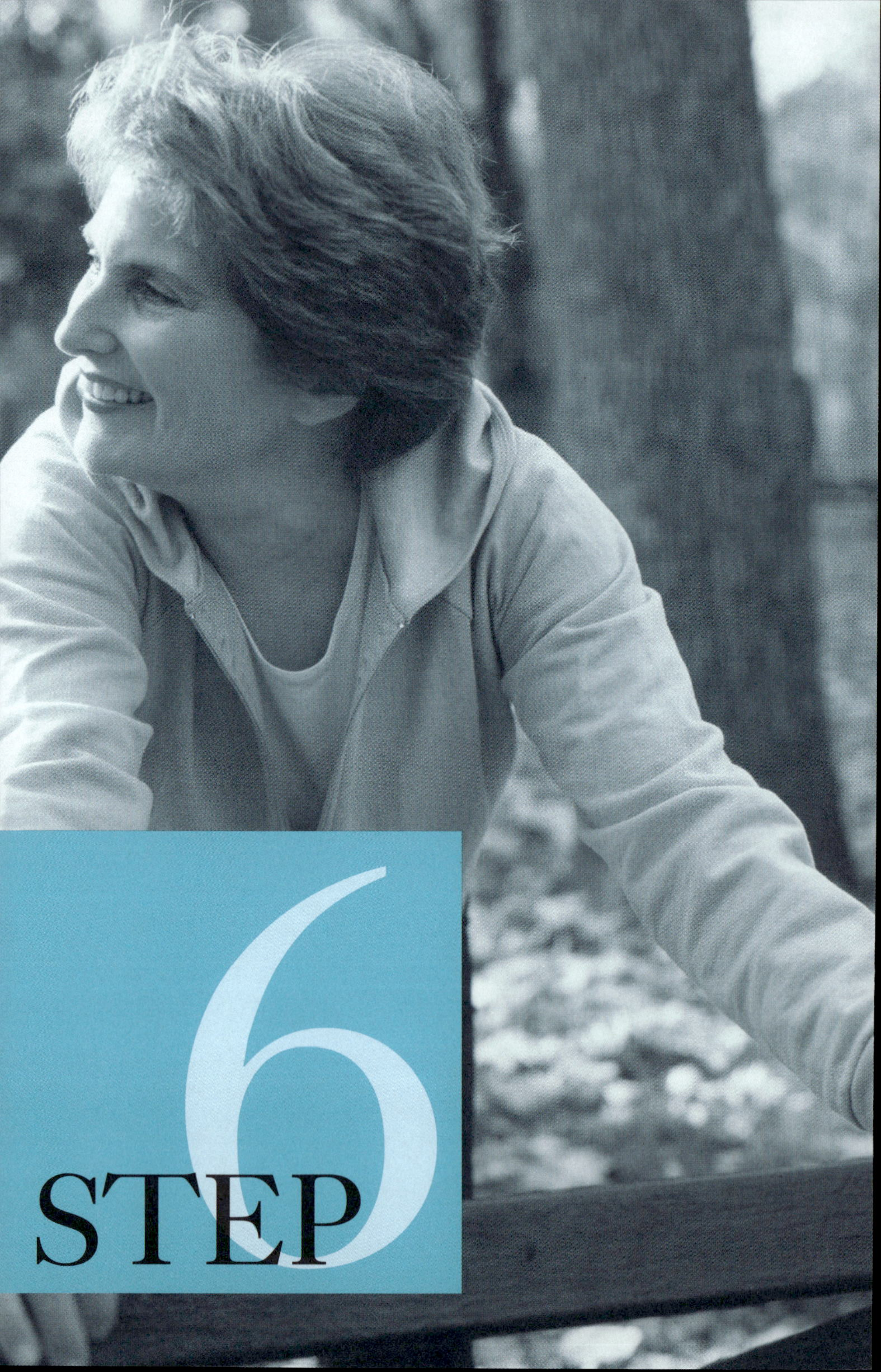

STEP 6

Respond immediately to red alerts

Most Australians tend to put off going to a GP. The first reactions to a new symptom are commonly: 'It'll go away.' 'I don't want to take up the doctor's time.' 'I'd rather not know.' As already discussed, some serious disorders are only picked up early with screening tests, but there are some symptoms and signs that you should never ignore. Early diagnosis and intervention can save your life.

The following illnesses have disabling complications. New technologies and medications are available to minimise these complications and prevent further recurrences. For example, most people who are treated early after a heart attack or stroke continue to lead a normal life. Many cancers can be cured. Early detection of diabetes, mental illness or osteoporosis can be treated with simple lifestyle changes. On the other hand, if these disorders are ignored or treated late, devastating effects can occur. Consult a GP immediately if you have any of the symptoms listed below.

'What I don't know won't hurt me. My body would let me know if something is going on but I don't run to the doctor with every little thing. There are a lot of hypochondriacs out there. I'm not one of them. I just keep a positive mind and everything will be OK.' Rebecca

Signs of heart disease

The first sign of heart pain can be exercise intolerance or breathlessness with exertion or at rest.

Any chest pain, but particularly chest pain, neck pain or arm pain, that increases with exercise or emotion and is relieved by rest is a medical emergency. If such chest pain occurs, immediately call an ambulance which will take you to the nearest accident and emergency centre at a local hospital.

Signs of stroke and other brain problems

Temporary or fleeting weakness, numbness or paralysis of the face, arm, leg, on either or both sides of the body can be signs of a mini stroke and should not be ignored. Lack of coordination is sometimes related to a dysfunction of the inner ear but may indicate a stroke or tumour in particular areas of the brain. Dizziness, loss of balance or an unexplained fall can also indicate a stroke.

Stroke and brain tumour may also manifest in unusual ways, such as:

- difficulty speaking or understanding
- loss of vision, sudden blurred or decreased vision in one or both eyes
- difficulty swallowing
- sudden memory, personality or behavioural changes.

Seizures are serious and should always be investigated with brain scans and electrical recordings.

Sudden severe headache can indicate rupture of weak blood vessels or aneurysms in the brain and immediate medical advice should be sought.

Some possible signs of cancer

There are many symptoms and signs which could indicate the possibility of cancer. If you experience any of these signs you should consult with your doctor. Some of the important symptoms and signs which should not be ignored include:

- Skin or mouth sores or ulcers that do not heal may indicate skin cancer or oral cancer.
- A change in a mole or a new mole or skin lesion could be the sign of a skin cancer.
- Unusual discharge or bleeding from the vagina is commonly a sign of infection but can also be cancer of the uterus. Vaginal bleeding in women who have finished menopause should always be investigated.
- An unexplained change in bowel function such as constipation or diarrhoea may indicate bowel cancer.
- Blood in the stools or on the paper after defecation can be due to rectal cancer.
- Blood in the urine may indicate bladder or kidney cancer.
- Persistent lower abdominal pain or feeling of abdominal fullness is commonly related to irritable bowel syndrome or diverticulitis, but may be a sign of cancer of one of the abdominal organs including ovary, bowel or pancreas.
- Unexplained loss of weight is commonly related to cancer or thyroid disease.
- A persistent lump in the breast, testis, neck, armpit, groin or other areas of the body should always be investigated for cancer.
- A persistent cough or coughing up blood may be related to lung cancer, particularly in smokers.
- Unexplained fever and fatigue can be caused by a number of different cancers including lymphoma.
- Persistent bone pain or spontaneous fracture may indicate bone cancer or secondary spread of malignancy.
- A persistent hoarse voice or the feeling of something sticking in the throat may be throat cancer.

- Anaemia may indicate underlying cancer of the stomach or bowel.
- Difficulty swallowing may be due to cancer of the oesophagus.
- Morning headache must be investigated to exclude brain tumour or high blood pressure.

Signs of mental illness and suicidal thinking

Depression is a serious condition and should be recognised early. Signs of depression include feeling sad most of the time, loss of interest or pleasure in normal activities, sleep disturbance, weight change, lack of energy, poor concentration, feelings of worthlessness, loss of libido (sex drive), generalised aches and pains, negative thinking and anxiety. Suicidal intent commonly manifests as feelings of hopelessness, overwhelming guilt, helplessness, withdrawal and isolation, sudden change in personality or strange behaviour and severe insomnia. Someone who is severely depressed and admits to having no plans for the future could be in an emergency situation as they may be planning a suicide.

Signs of dementia

Early signs of dementia can be subtle and include progressive loss of memory, confusion, loss of ability to carry out everyday activities and change in personality.

Signs of diabetes

Persistent thirst and fatigue, frequency of urine, including urinating at night and recurrent infections such as boils or thrush are common signs of diabetes. However, early diabetes is often silent.

Signs of kidney disease

Kidney disease often has few symptoms until it becomes very serious. Symptoms may include changes in frequency of urine, blood in the urine, pain in the back, swelling and puffiness of ankles and face. As the kidneys fail, people may develop symptoms of tiredness, nausea, shortness of breath, loss of appetite and feeling generally unwell.

Signs of osteoporosis

Osteoporosis is often silent but sometimes presents as an easy bone fracture, changes in posture, muscle weakness, loss of height and hunchback or chronic back pain. If you stub your toe and find it's still sore after a few weeks, it may be best to have it X-rayed to confirm any fracture. It's also important to see your GP if you gradually lose over three centimetres in height compared with your peak height measurement at age 21.

Signs of glaucoma

Visual loss due to glaucoma may be sudden and painful or gradual, leading to permanent blindness if not treated early.

These are just some of the warning symptoms and signs of possible serious disease. If you have any worrying symptoms please consult your GP. It could save your life.

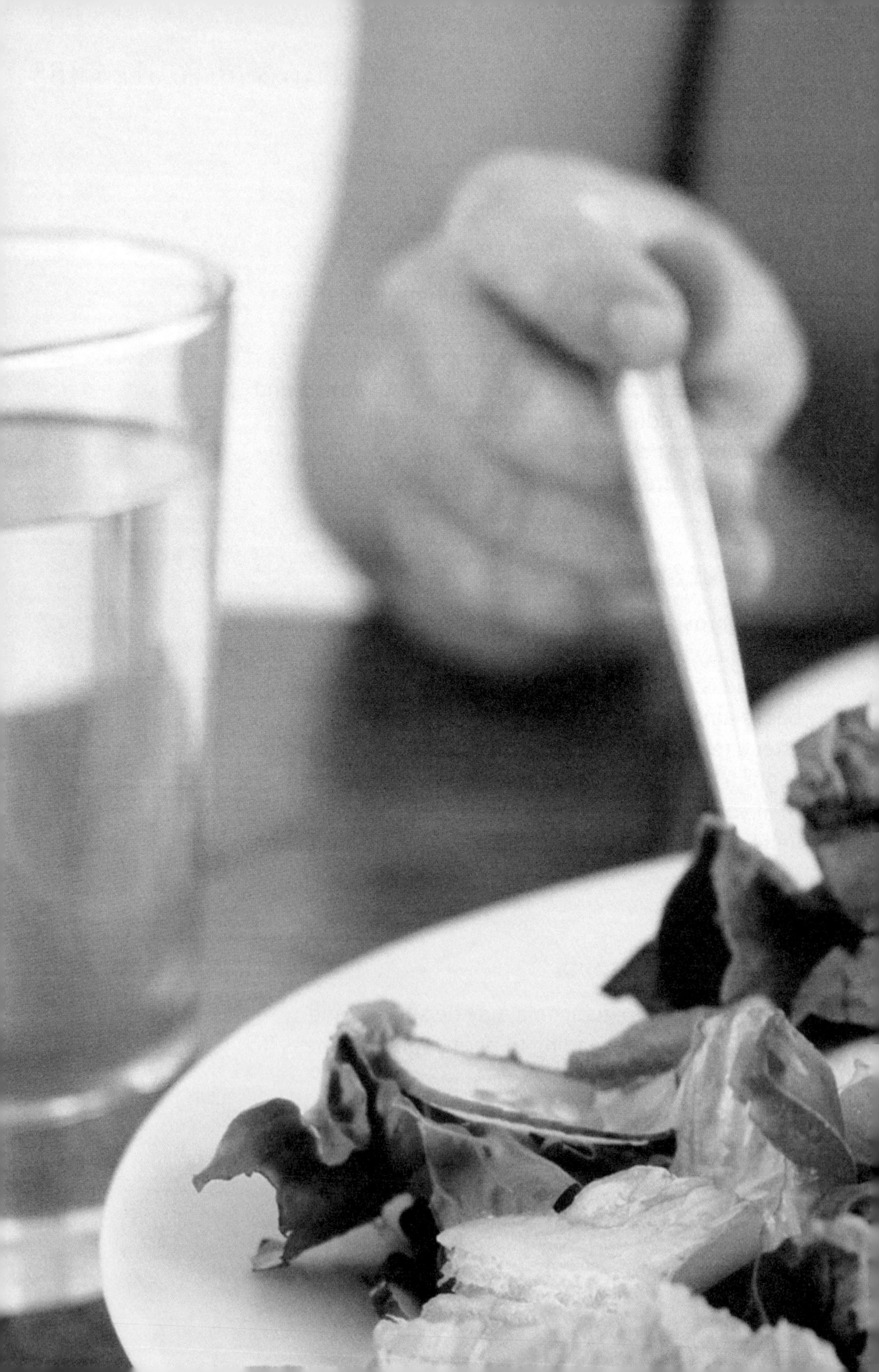

PART TWO

THE BIG NINE: HOW TO PREVENT AND TREAT COMMON LIFE THREATENING ILLNESSES

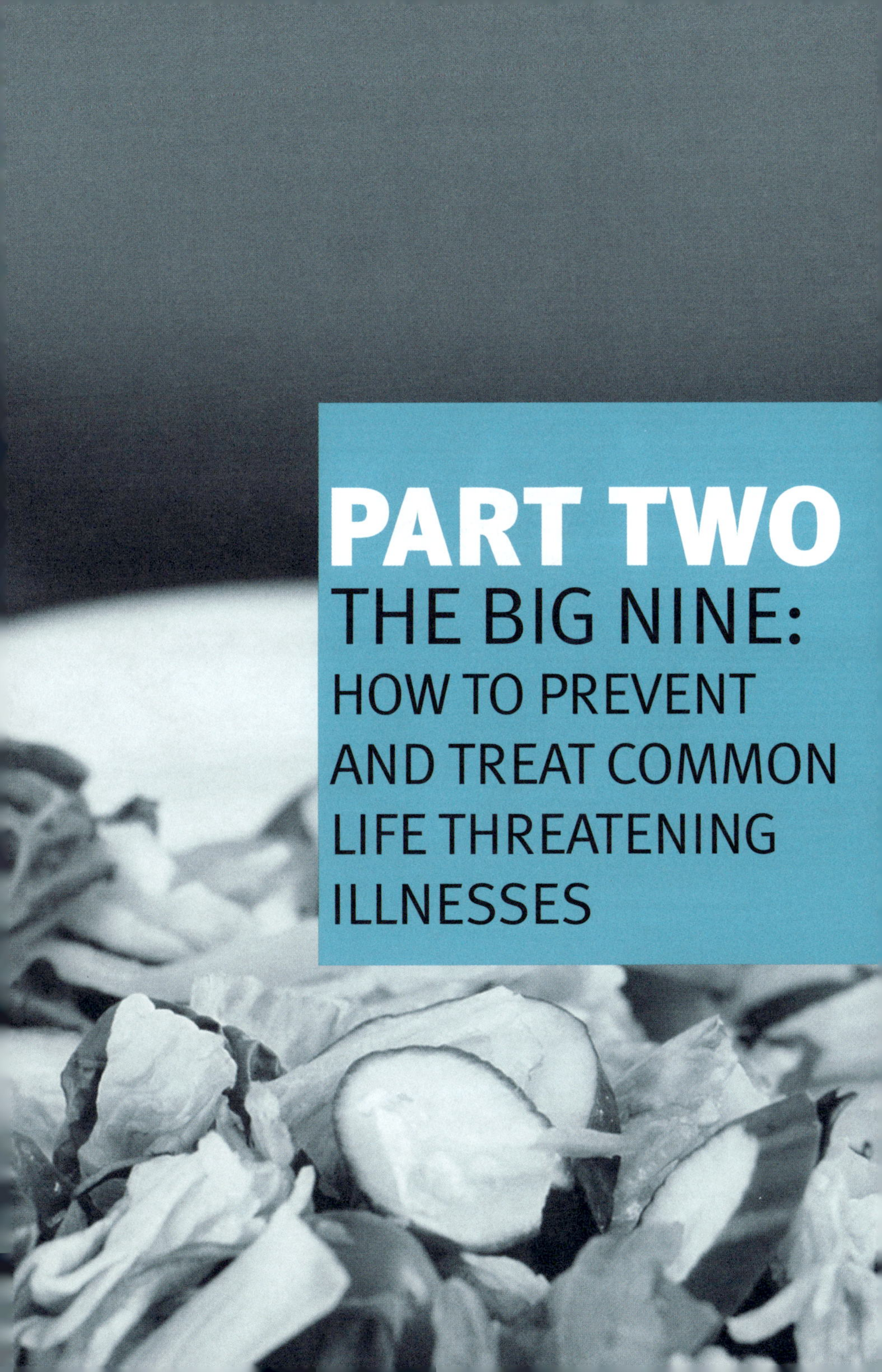

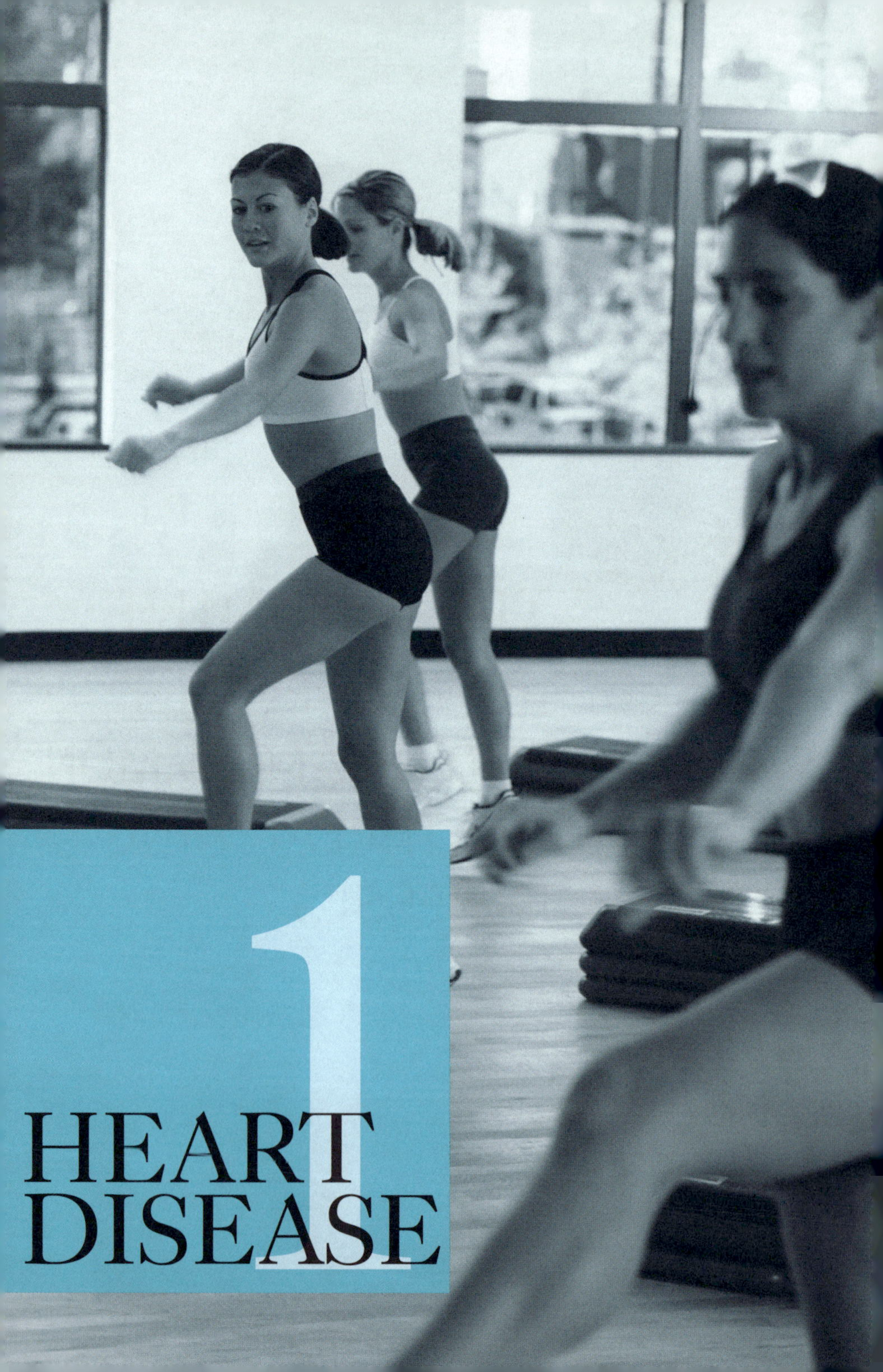

1 HEART DISEASE

Heart disease

Despite advances in enormously expensive health technology to treat heart disease, its prevalence is increasing. About 3.4 million Australians have a long-term circulatory disorder and heart disease accounts for 18 per cent of all deaths. With a healthy lifestyle and regular health screening, you can prevent a lot of the causes of heart disease and heart attack. It is surprising that despite the devastating nature of heart attack most people do not change their lifestyle, even after a cardiac event.

fast facts

The cost of heart disease to our community is about $4400 million per year.

The most common form of heart disease results from a build-up of fatty deposits in the arteries that supply the heart (the coronary arteries). The fatty deposits start in childhood and gradually cause a narrowing of your arteries, blocking the supply of blood flow, oxygen and nutrients to your heart. A heart attack occurs when a narrowed coronary artery is suddenly blocked by a blood clot. This is a life threatening medical emergency because medical or surgical treatment is required to restore the blood flow and to prevent permanent heart muscle damage.

Angina is the heart pain or discomfort related to narrowed coronary arteries and temporary lack of

'I'd been going to the gym three to four times a week for years, but this time I had a feeling like someone was squeezing my chest tight and I couldn't breathe for a few minutes. I put the pain in my left shoulder down to a stretched muscle. When I did see the doctor he ordered a stress test, which I failed dismally. An angiogram showed that I had a 92 per cent blockage of my main artery to my heart. I suddenly found myself waiting for a bypass.

I am 48. I wasn't the type to go to the doctor. Now I would recommend for everyone to have a regular check-up. I have learnt the hard way that women can have heart disease too.' Belinda

blood supply to the heart muscle. The pain of angina usually occurs when you exercise and resolves with rest. It is a symptom of coronary heart disease.

Who is at risk?

Heart and blood vessel disease is the leading cause of death and disability in our society. About 3.4 million people are affected by circulatory disease.

Despite all the advances in treatment of heart disease, the prevalence has increased by 18.2 per cent in the last decade. Males are two to three times more likely to die of heart disease than women. For a 40 year old, the future risk of heart disease is one in two for men and one in three for women. The difference between male and female life expectancy is due largely to the increased risk of heart disease in males. Women should not be reassured by this statistic: heart disease still kills more than 12 000 Australian women each year—almost five times the number for breast cancer.

RISK QUIZ FOR HEART DISEASE

DO YOU HAVE ANY OF THE FOLLOWING RISK FACTORS?		
Smoking	Yes	No
Low physical activity	Yes	No
High blood pressure	Yes	No
Obesity	Yes	No
High cholesterol	Yes	No
Diabetes	Yes	No
Family history of heart disease or sudden cardiac death	Yes	No
Depression, social isolation and lack of social support	Yes	No
Obstructive sleep apnoea	Yes	No

RED ALERT!!!!

If you experience early signs of exercise intolerance or breathlessness with exertion it may signal partial blockage of the arteries supplying the heart. Angina usually presents as central chest pain, neck pain or arm pain that increases with exercise or emotion and is relieved by rest. Do not confuse these symptoms with indigestion, which is usually related to meals. Call an ambulance and proceed directly to the nearest accident and emergency centre if you have any doubt.

CONTINUED

If you answered 'Yes' to any of these questions you must undergo screening tests for BMI, blood pressure, cholesterol and urine tests for protein, in your early forties or earlier.

To calculate your individual risk of developing heart disease, refer to the New Zealand Guidelines Cardiovascular Risk Calculator <www.nzgg.org.nz/guidelines/0035/cvd_risk_chart.pdf>.

If heart disease is not prevented or treated and the pumping action of your heart is affected by extensive damage to your muscle cells, sudden death or heart failure may result. Heart failure may be mild, moderate or severe and is usually permanent and disabling but it can be alleviated with lifelong medication. Heart failure symptoms are chronic fatigue, breathlessness, chest pain and swelling of the abdomen and ankles.

How can you prevent heart disease?

Heart disease can be prevented and treated by addressing the risk factors including:

- smoking (Step 5)
- inactivity (Step 4)
- high blood pressure (Step 1)
- obesity (Step 3)
- high cholesterol (Step 1)
- diabetes (Chapter 7)
- obstructive sleep apnoea (this chapter).

Good nutrition and adequate exercise remain your best protection against this sometimes silent killer. Fish oil to reduce the chance of sudden death from heart disease is very beneficial. If you are at high risk of heart disease or have existing heart disease,

RED ALERT!!!!

A heart attack often presents as a severe crushing pain in the centre of your chest or behind your breastbone. This may be a squeezing, tightening, choking or heavy pressure feeling. The pain may spread or start in your shoulders, arms, neck, throat or jaw and may be associated with sweating, dizziness, nausea, shortness of breath or collapse. Go directly by ambulance to the nearest accident and emergency centre if you experience any of these symptoms.

low-dose aspirin may be used to prevent future cardiac events. Aspirin has been shown to reduce heart attack by about 30 per cent but it can be associated with bleeding from the gastrointestinal tract or the brain. Your main defence is diet and exercise.

Diet

The type of fat you eat is important for your health not only in relation to your weight. A diet high in saturated fat increases your blood LDL (the 'unhealthy' cholesterol), which clogs arteries with fatty plaques, even in people who are underweight. Foods high in saturated fat include:

- meat fat and offal (such as kidney, liver, brains)
- full-fat dairy foods (such as milk, cheese, butter, ice-cream, cream)
- solid cooking fats (such as butter, lard, copha and ghee)
- oils (such as palm and coconut, and products that contain these fats, for example pastries, fried foods, potato crisps, corn crisps, cakes, chocolate, biscuits, toasted muesli and many snack, packaged and junk foods).

Some foods are high in cholesterol, including shellfish and egg yolk. However, the cholesterol you take in your diet through these sources has less effect on blood levels of LDL cholesterol than saturated fat.

Meat and dairy products are promoted in some high-protein weight-loss diets. As discussed under Step 3 these diets may help you to reduce weight in the short term, but in the long term they can lead to increased risk of heart disease if high in saturated fat. Dried peas, beans and lentils are healthier sources of protein, but excessive amounts are unpalatable, poor sources of energy and wind producing. We recommend that you include a balance of trim meat, low-fat dairy and vegetable sources of protein in your diet.

Polyunsaturated fats and oils

Polyunsaturated fats and oils reduce the risk of heart disease by lowering the LDL in the blood. They are found in:

- polyunsaturated margarines
- sunflower, safflower, soybean, corn, cottonseed, grape seed and sesame oils
- oily fish such as herring, mackerel, sardine, salmon and tuna
- nuts and seeds.

Omega-3 polyunsaturated fats are found predominantly in fish. If you eat fish at least twice a week you are less likely to die from heart disease because omega-3 polyunsaturated fats lower triglyceride levels and protect against clotting in diseased blood vessels. Intake of fish oil has been proven to reduce the risk of cardiac death in people with heart disease. Another polyunsaturated fat, alpha linolenic acid, is found in canola and soybean oils and it also lowers your cholesterol and reduces your risk of heart disease.

Mono-unsaturated fats and oils

Mono-unsaturated fats and oils, such as canola or olive oil margarines, canola and olive oil, avocados, nuts and seeds, have also been shown to lower LDL cholesterol but not to the same extent as polyunsaturated fats.

MARGARINE VERSUS BUTTER

Many Australians have switched from butter to margarines made of polyunsaturated and mono-unsaturated oils; however, the public perception that margarine is less fattening than butter is wrong. Margarine has the same high-calorie level and fat content as butter. Margarine does have lower saturated fat content than butter but, if you use margarine, you will not necessarily reduce heart disease as margarine still contains about 25 per cent of saturated fat (butter contains about 60 per cent saturated fat). Less or no margarine or butter is probably the healthier choice.

Trans fats

Trans fats are a type of hydrogenated fat which raises LDL and lowers HDL (the good cholesterol), and are very effective at clogging your arteries. These fats are produced when vegetable oils are hydrogenated to produce margarine and deep frying oils, and are mostly found in biscuits and pastries. Most margarines in Australia are produced with very low levels of trans fats (less than 1 per cent).

Spreads made with plant sterols

Spreads made with plant sterols have about 50 per cent less fat than butter or margarine. An intake of two to three grams per day (or one to one and a half tablespoons) of plant sterol-enriched margarine reduces cholesterol by 10 per cent. These margarines are not suitable for pregnant women, children, or for use in cooking as they deplete betacarotene and other carotenoids in your body, substances that protect your eyes and have anti-cancer properties. If you switch to margarine made with plant sterols, you will need to eat more yellow and orange vegetables to make up for these depleted substances. No studies have been conducted on the long-term effects of plant sterols.

Wholegrains

Wholegrains lower the risk of heart disease. Dietary fibre in wholegrains, oats, barley, psyllium and legumes also lower blood cholesterol levels. Experts recommend that you eat about 20 to 30 grams of fibre each day including at least 6 grams of wholegrain fibre. This amount of fibre can be obtained by eating seven serves of fruit and vegetables and wholegrain breakfast cereals and bread each day. Dietary fibre as an energy value per gram is 13 kilojoules. You may find a high-fibre diet based on legumes, wholegrain breads and cereals, vegetables and fruit very bland. Herbs, rather than salt and processed sauces, are a great way to make food more interesting.

Reduce salt

You should limit your salt intake to less than 2.3 grams per day (less than 6 grams of table salt or one and a half teaspoons) as it has an adverse effect on blood pressure and therefore heart disease. High levels of salt are found in rock salt, garlic salt, bread, meat paste, fish paste, tomato paste, commercial sauces, tomato sauce, salad dressing, pickles, olives, soup powders, packet seasonings, stock cubes, bacon, ham and breakfast cereals. Most of your daily salt however may come from processed foods that do not actually taste salty, including biscuits, cheese, bread and processed cereals like cornflakes.

Increase potassium

Potassium lowers blood pressure. Food sources of potassium include fruits and vegetables, unsalted nuts, dried peas, dried beans and lentils. Food processing tends to lower potassium and increase salt content in many foods. Therefore it is better to eat unprocessed foods such as wholegrain breads and cereals.

Alcohol

Some studies show a benefit of drinking a moderate amount of red wine. In these studies, women who drank one glass of red wine a day and men who drank two glasses of red wine a day had a lower risk of heart attack in middle age.

Obstructive sleep apnoea

Obstructive sleep apnoea is a disorder of breathing during sleep, usually meaning the person alternates between snoring and breath holding. This disorder is associated with heart disease, heart failure, sudden cardiac death and stroke. It may be treated by losing weight, quitting smoking and avoiding alcohol and other sedatives. Continuous positive airway pressure (CPAP) is sometimes required to treat obstructive sleep apnoea. It consists of a face mask attached to a machine, which blows pressurized air into the mask and through your airways to keep these open. One of the immediate results of treatment for obstructive sleep apnoea is relief of fatigue.

What are the treatments?

There are many new treatments for angina, heart disease and heart attack, including complex medications, cardiac catheterisation and stents to keep coronary arteries open, cardiac bypass, where the coronary arteries are replaced, and even heart transplant. Many of these interventions are risky and carry with them serious side effects. If you adopt simple lifestyle changes to prevent heart disease you will find it is a much better and easier strategy. If you are at risk of heart disease or have heart disease you may benefit from increasing your intake of fish oil and the regular use of low-dose aspirin.

The Australian Resuscitation Council has recently issued new guidelines on management of cardiac arrest (<www.resus.org.au>). This organisation provides training on cardiopulmonary resuscitation, which is an important skill for every Australian to learn. The basic steps include checking for danger, monitoring responsiveness and calling 000 (or 112 on a mobile telephone) for an ambulance. The guidelines state: if there are no signs of life, open the airway, give two initial breaths, followed by 30 central chest compressions. Continue this cycle at a rate of about two compressions a second until assistance arrives.

TAKE AWAY MESSAGE

Heart disease is common, deadly and costly, but preventable. All healthy people should be screened for cholesterol from the age of 45 and for blood pressure from the age of 18. If you have a family history or other risk factors, you should be screened for cholesterol earlier and more frequently.

If you ever experience central chest pain, radiating to the neck or left arm, which is not relieved by rest, go immediately to your closest accident and emergency centre by ambulance. Unfortunately many people confuse heart attack with indigestion and die without early treatment.

For general information on heart health, talk to your GP or call the Heart Foundation's Heartline. Heartline is a dedicated telephone service answered by qualified health professionals, providing information and support on any aspect of heart health and surgery.

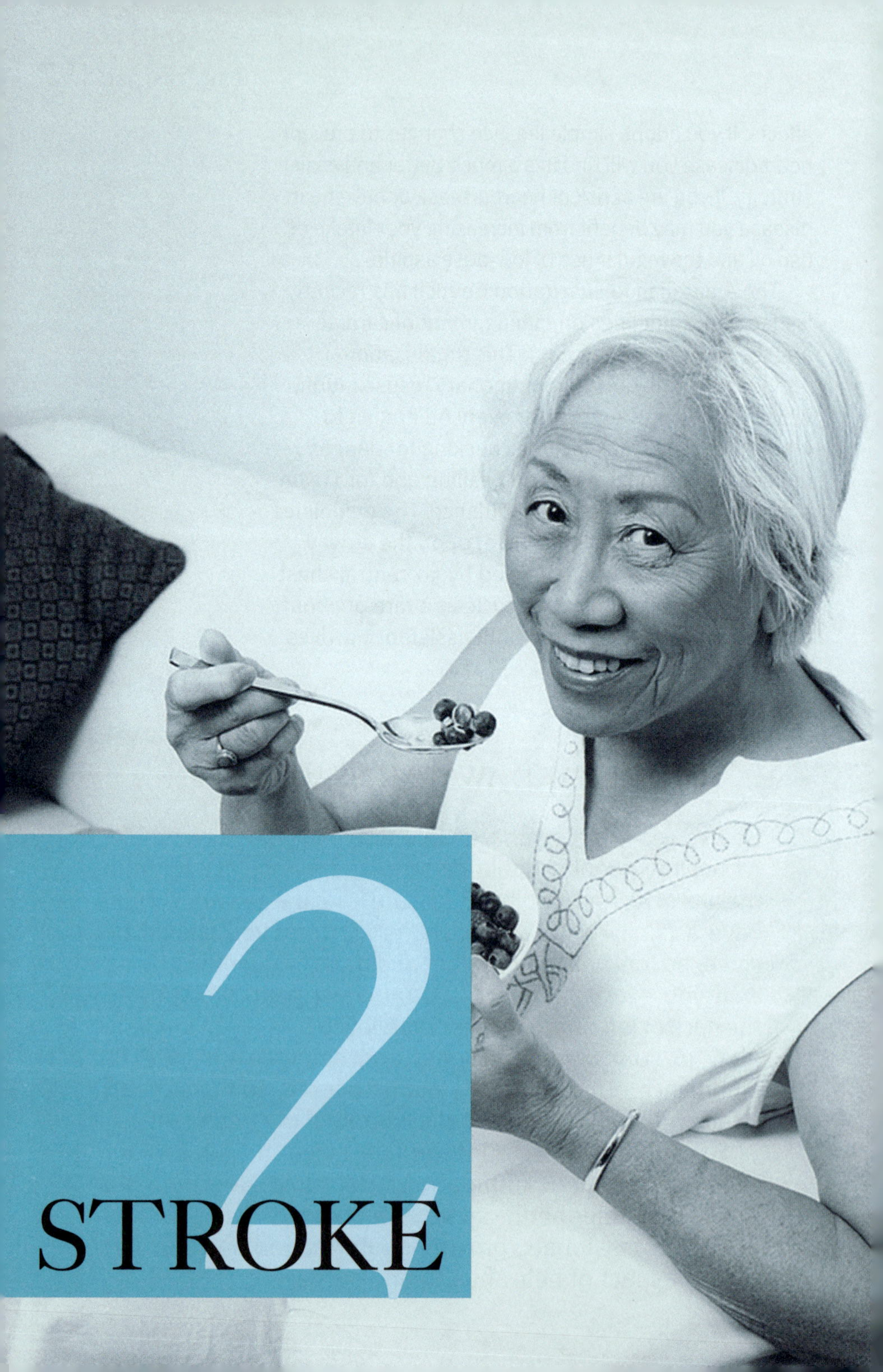

2 STROKE

Stroke

fast facts

About 48 000 Australians suffer stroke each year. Young people also suffer strokes—about 2000 strokes occur in people aged under 45 years in Australia each year. Stroke accounts for about 8600 deaths each year and is more common in women. Stroke costs the community up to $2 billion annually, including about $1 billion in direct health costs.

Stroke is a sudden brain injury caused by narrowing, blockage or rupture of the blood vessels to your brain. It is Australia's third biggest killer after heart disease and cancer and causes approximately 10 per cent of all deaths and 25 per cent of chronic disability in our community.

Despite the devastating nature of stroke, most people ignore early warning signs. Symptoms such as transient facial weakness, or temporary blindness are a medical emergency.

Unfortunately many Australians who have had a stroke fail to prevent a recurrence of stroke by ignoring their risk factors or forgetting to take their preventive medication. Blood pressure, cholesterol and anticoagulant treatment need careful monitoring after stroke.

‘I remember feeling some weakness down my right side while I was driving. Somehow I managed to make it to my father's house and he called an ambulance. It took months to recover and it's been difficult to take this amount of time off work and not being able to support my young family—I'm only 35. I am now on tablets for high blood pressure. If I had known that everyone over 18 was meant to have their blood pressure checked every two years, maybe my stroke would have been prevented.’ Ramesh

Who is at risk?

You are at a higher risk of stroke if you have:

- Abnormal electrical activity in the heart known as atrial fibrillation (irregular electrical activity in the heart causing pounding or fluttering of the heart, palpitations, dizziness, faintness or light-headedness and sometimes chest pain), which is more common in people over 65 and also in people who have heart or thyroid disease. Atrial fibrillation can be confirmed by an electrocardiograph.
- Transient neurological symptoms suggestive of a mini stroke (transient ischaemic attack), such as temporary neurological symptoms—dizzy spells or 'funny turns'—weakness or numbness of arms or legs, speech disturbance, double vision or vertigo.
- A past history of heart attack or diabetes.

RISK QUIZ FOR STROKE

DO YOU HAVE ANY OF THE FOLLOWING RISK FACTORS?		
High blood pressure	Yes	No
High cholesterol	Yes	No
Smoking	Yes	No
Excessive alcohol intake	Yes	No
Obesity	Yes	No
Low physical activity	Yes	No
Diabetes	Yes	No
History of a transient ischaemic attack	Yes	No
History of atrial fibrillation	Yes	No

If you answered 'Yes' to any of the questions above, you may be at risk of stroke and you must be screened regularly by a GP for early warning signs of stroke.

RED ALERT!!!!

Many strokes have warning signs due to temporary interruptions to the blood supply to the brain and therefore can be prevented from worsening. Never ignore signs of a stroke that disappear after a short period. See a doctor immediately if you experience anything that resembles signs of a transient ischaemic attack including:

- weakness, numbness or paralysis of the face or an arm or leg on either or both sides of the body
- lack of coordination
- difficulty

CONTINUED

How can you prevent stroke?

Stroke may cause sudden, permanent disability or death. Of those who suffer a stroke, one third will die within the first 12 months, one third will be disabled and one third will recover. You can prevent stroke if you modify your risk factors, such as high blood pressure, high cholesterol, smoking, obesity, inactivity and diabetes (Steps 1, 3 and 4, Chapter 7).

A number of studies have shown that one or two standard glasses of red wine a day may protect you from stroke. However, excessive alcohol can raise blood pressure, thereby increasing the risk of stroke. Your doctor may recommend treatment with aspirin or blood-thinning medication (anticoagulants) as a preventive measure if you have risk factors, such as atrial fibrillation and/or transient ischaemic attack.

What are the treatments?

Stroke is always a medical emergency. Without prompt medical treatment brain damage may be permanent and disabling. There are many advances in the treatment of stroke that prevent further brain damage. These treatments may be medications or surgical interventions, such as a carotid endarterectomy, to unclog arteries. Carotid endarterectomy is usually performed if there is over 70 per cent of stenosis (abnormal narrowing of the blood vessel) in a carotid artery. Rehabilitation after stroke can be a long haul but often results in very good outcomes.

RED ALERT!!!!

speaking or understanding

- dizziness, loss of balance or an unexplained fall
- loss of vision, sudden blurred or decreased vision in one or both eyes
- difficulty swallowing
- memory, personality or behavioural changes
- seizures.

A stroke is a permanent blockage of the blood vessels of your brain and causes prolonged or permanent neurological signs. Rupture of weak blood vessels or aneurysms in the brain usually also result in sudden severe headache.

TAKE AWAY MESSAGE

Control of stroke risk factors and early detection can greatly reduce your chances of having a stroke. Make sure your 'numbers', including your blood pressure, cholesterol and BMI, are monitored regularly and are normal, particularly if you have a family history of stroke.

Stroke is always a medical emergency. Call an ambulance immediately and proceed to the nearest accident and emergency centre. Without prompt medical treatment brain damage can occur and it may be permanent and disabling.

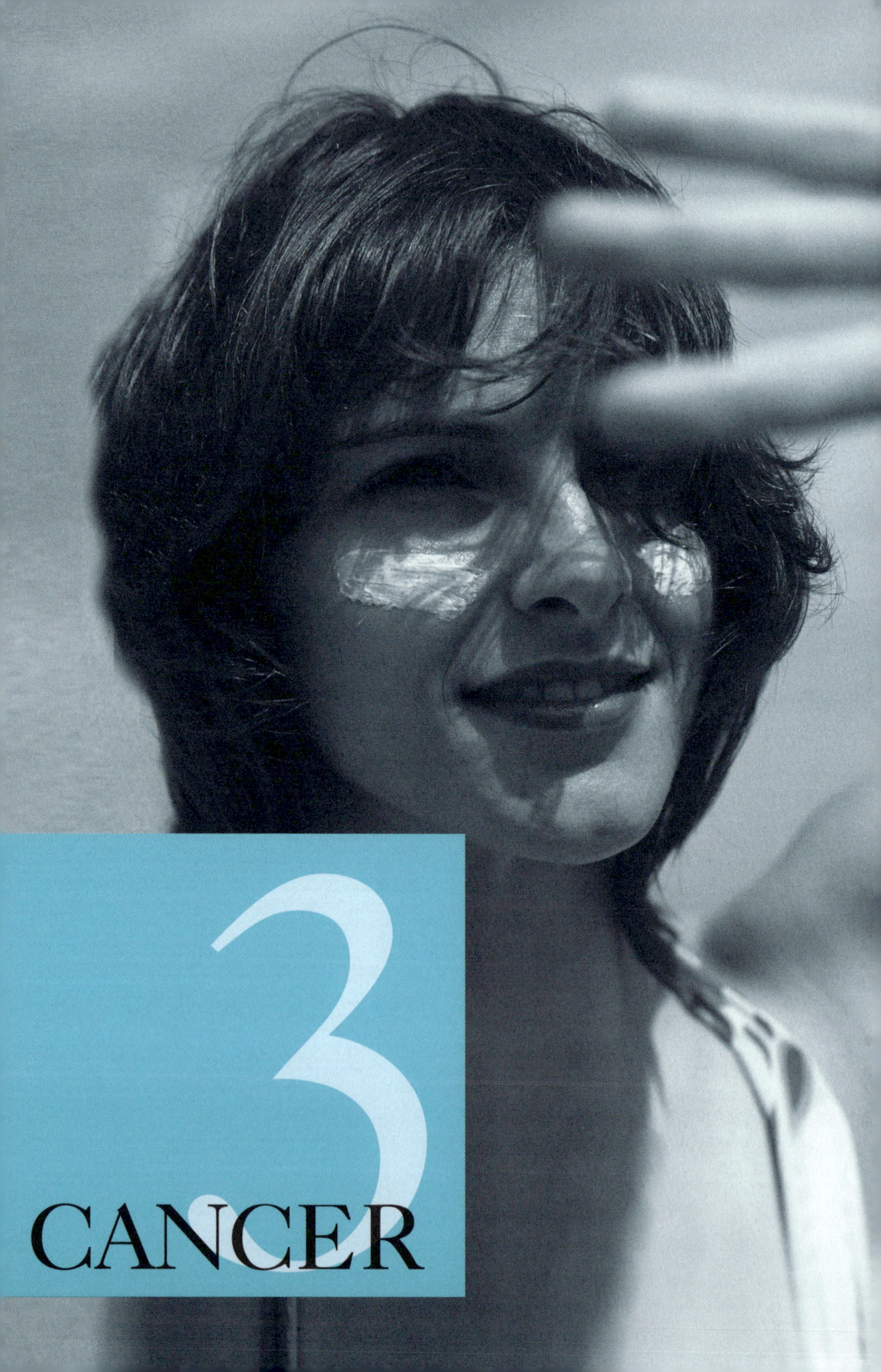

3
CANCER

Cancer

fast facts

One in three men and one in four women will be directly affected by cancer before the age of 75.

Cancer costs $3.8 billion in direct health system costs each year in Australia.

Cancer is now the leading cause of death in Australians aged 45 to 64. About 40 000 Australians die from cancer each year. Much of the burden of cancer can be prevented or cured if diagnosed early, particularly in the case of prostate cancer, breast cancer, bowel cancer, skin cancer and cervical cancer. Prostate, breast, bowel, skin and cervical cancers are covered in detail in this chapter because they are common cancers that can be diagnosed early with screening and treated successfully.

‘Many people fear cancer and live in denial. Cancer is a word, not a sentence. It's important to actively prevent cancer and when it does occur to diagnose it early. New treatments are becoming available all the time for different forms of cancer. There is a lot of hope and optimism—many cancers can be cured.’ Daniel

What is cancer?

Cancer occurs when cells in your body grow in an uncontrolled way. A malignant tumour is a lump of these abnormal cells. If these cells are not treated, they spread to other tissues and affect the function of major body organs. Each year, more than 104 000 new cases of cancer are diagnosed in Australia. More than half of them will be successfully treated. The survival rate for many common cancers has increased by more than 30 per cent in the past two decades.

RED ALERT!!!!

Warning signs of cancer may include sores or ulcers that do not heal, unusual discharge or bleeding, unexplained changes in bowel or bladder function, unexplained loss of weight, a lump in the breast, neck, armpit or other areas of the body, a persistent cough or a change to an existing mole or a new mole. If you are worried about a change in your body, see your GP without delay.

The most common cancers in Australia (excluding non-melanoma skin cancers) are:

- colorectal (bowel)
- breast
- prostate
- melanoma (skin)
- lung.

Lung cancer is most commonly related to smoking (Step 5), is nearly always diagnosed late (only 12 per cent of people diagnosed with lung cancer survive more than five years) and results in over 7000 deaths a year. It is covered in more detail in Chapter 4 under lung disease.

Nutrition and cancer

You are more likely to protect yourself from cancer if you eat seven or more serves of vegetables, fruit, grain products and legumes each day. The strongest protective anti-cancer effect has been shown with:

- vegetables, especially raw vegetables or salads
- leafy green vegetables
- cruciferous vegetables, like broccoli, cabbage, brussels sprouts, bok choy and other Asian greens
- carrots
- tomatoes
- citrus fruits.

To help prevent cancer, also try to avoid low-fibre foods and highly processed starchy foods. The less processed the grains the better, as diets high in refined starch and refined sugar may increase your risk of stomach or bowel cancer.

Current evidence does not indicate a direct link between fat intake and any types of cancer with the possible exception of prostate cancer. However, a high-fat diet may lead to obesity and obesity is a risk factor for several cancers. Similarly, cured meats (such as bacon, ham, salami and smoked meats) have not been shown to be directly related to cancer, but it is best for you to limit the amount of cured meats in your diet because they are generally high in fat and salt. Salt has also been associated with an increased risk of stomach cancer and should be consumed in limited amounts.

A group of carcinogenic substances called 'polycyclic aromatic hydrocarbons' (PAHs) can be produced if foods are overheated or burnt. While it has not been proven that chargrilled meats and foods cause cancer, it is probably best for you to use relatively low-temperature cooking methods, such as steaming, boiling, poaching, stewing, casserolling, braising, baking or stir-frying; microwaving; or roasting and cooking meat until golden rather than brown or black.

Antioxidants are substances that may protect against cancer. The best source of antioxidants is fresh food including fresh fruits, vegetables and wholegrain cereals. These foods are better alternatives to taking supplements.

Artificial sweeteners including saccharin and cyclamate are used as sugar substitutes to sweeten foods and beverages. There is no clear evidence that artificial sweeteners are related to cancer risk in humans.

Recent international research has suggested that regular tea drinking can slow down certain cancers and reduce the risk of diseases such as heart disease. If you drink green tea rather than black tea you may give yourself more protection against cancer.

PROSTATE CANCER

'One of the things that made me concerned was that my dad had it. My urine stream was getting weaker and my prostate blood test was climbing each year. My urologist put an instrument in my rear passage and took eight samples of prostate tissue, four of which were positive. I opted for surgical treatment, having my prostate removed. I knew there were other options like radiotherapy but I've kept this up my sleeve in case the cancer returns. I was in intensive care for three days after the surgery with tubes coming out of everywhere, but now I've made a complete recovery with no side effects.' Ben

Prostate cancer occurs when abnormal prostate cells grow out of control. The prostate cancer cells eventually break out of the prostate and invade distant parts of the body, producing secondary tumours, a process known as metastasis. Early treatment is more likely to have a better outcome. Every year, over 17 000 Australian men are diagnosed and nearly 3000 die of the disease, making prostate cancer the second largest cause of male cancer deaths, after lung cancer. As many men die of prostate cancer as women die of breast cancer.

fast facts

Prostate cancer is the third most common cause of death of men in Australia, affecting one in 11 men, commonly over 65 years of age.

Who is at risk?

The exact causes of prostate cancer are unknown; however, your chance of getting prostate cancer increases with age and family history. A high saturated-fat intake in your diet may put you at greater risk.

What are the warning signs?

Early prostate cancer usually causes no symptoms. When symptoms do occur, they may include:

- difficulties starting and stopping urination
- pain or a burning sensation when passing urine

- urinating more often than usual, particularly at night
- the feeling that the bladder can't be fully emptied
- dribbling urine
- blood in the urine or semen
- pain during ejaculation.

All of these symptoms can also be caused by conditions other than prostate cancer. You should discuss them with your GP as soon as you notice any one of the symptoms.

How can you prevent prostate cancer?

Recent research suggests a low-fat diet that includes fish, vegetables, fruit, wholegrains, legumes, lycopenes (found in cooked tomatoes, tomato sauces and ketchup) and exercise, may prevent prostate cancer. Other research suggests these lifestyle interventions may not only prevent but may also help arrest progression of prostate cancer.

When to have a screening test

Routine screening is currently not recommended because the tests tend to be unreliable and the treatments invasive. However, all men should be aware of the potential risks, benefits and uncertainties of screening for prostate cancer so they can make an individual choice based on their level of risk, particularly if there is a family history of prostate cancer.

Prostate cancer is diagnosed using a number of tests, which may include a PSA test and digital rectal examination by your GP.

Digital rectal examination

Your GP can feel for enlargement and irregularities of your prostate by examining inside your anus with a gloved finger.

PSA test

The prostate makes a protein called prostate specific antigen (PSA), which can be found in your blood via a simple blood test. However, this test may be unreliable. Cancer can still be present with a normal PSA test. Alternatively, PSA can be elevated if you have a benign enlargement of the prostate, urinary infection or retention, or an inflammation of the prostate, and after you ejaculate. The normal range for the level of PSA depends on your age. If your PSA is abnormal, you may be retested three to six months later, before a biopsy is considered.The question remains about what to do with a borderline or even an abnormal PSA test.

A biopsy of the prostate involves twelve tissue samples taken from the prostate under ultrasound guidance and examined in a laboratory for the presence of cancer cells. A biopsy of the prostate is not to be taken lightly as it may result in problems with infection and sexual function.

It is important for you to understand the complexity of the management of prostate cancer before you make a decision about prostate cancer testing. Ultimately this choice depends on whether you would prefer:

1. **'To know if you had prostate cancer'** and for you to be involved in making decisions about early treatment of prostate cancer because of the chance of cure without long term complication,

particularly if your tumour is aggressive or life threatening; or

2. **'Not to know if you had prostate cancer'** in view of the uncertainties about testing and the risks of complications associated with surgery and other treatments, especially for harmless or slow-growing tumours.

The choice is yours. Your GP will assist you to make an informed choice.

What are the treatments?

Prostate cancer is usually one of the slower-growing cancers. After diagnosis the majority of men survive for ten years or more. In the past, prostate cancer tended to be a disease in men over 70 years of age, and they were more likely to die of other causes before the cancer could kill them. As men are living longer these days, prostate cancer in older men is more likely to spread and cause complications. More recently there has been a reported increase in aggressive forms of prostate cancer in men younger than 50.

Treatments for prostate cancer can affect your quality of life and need to be considered carefully. About 12 per cent of men suffer with incontinence and up to 66 per cent of men suffer with erectile dysfunction about three years after a radical prostatectomy. While the side effects of prostate surgery are serious, a number of newer treatments, such as a highly accurate form of radiotherapy called brachytherapy, and high-intensity focused ultrasound, are less likely to damage the surrounding tissues than surgery and also offer a chance of cure.

TAKE AWAY MESSAGE

Prostate cancer is increasing in incidence with over 17 000 new prostate cancers diagnosed in Australia every year. There are as many deaths in men from prostate cancer as in women from breast cancer.

If you wish to be tested, talk with your GP.

Prostate surgery has serious side effects but new techniques and follow-up treatment are showing more promise. It is important for men to understand their treatment options, along with the importance of diet and exercise in preventing prostate cancer.

BREAST CANCER

Breast cancer occurs when abnormal breast cells grow out of control. It is the most common type of cancer in women in the world. In Australia, there are over 12 600 women diagnosed each year. Breast cancer affects one in 11 Australian women, commonly over the age of 50 years.

fast facts

Although breast cancer cases are increasing, the survival rate for women diagnosed with breast cancer is improving. Eighty-five per cent of women survive more than five years after being diagnosed with breast cancer.

Who is at risk?

About 70 per cent of breast cancer is diagnosed in women without any risk factors. The exact cause of breast cancer is unknown, but major risk factors include:

- gender—being a woman (while extremely rare, men can develop breast cancer—refer to <www.breasthealth.com.au/men>)
- age—most cases occur in women over 50
- family history, especially if two or more close relatives—mother, sister or daughter—have had breast or ovarian cancer and/or if one or two close relatives were younger than 50 when their cancer was diagnosed
- previous history of breast cancer—women who have had breast cancer have a greater risk of developing it again
- genetic—if you are a member of a family that has the high-risk breast cancer gene mutation.

Only a very small number of women have an increased risk of breast cancer by having an inherited gene. Two genes called BRCA 1 and BRCA 2 help prevent breast cancer. When these genes are abnormal, women have a higher chance of developing breast cancer. However, most breast cancers occur by chance.

There are a number of other factors associated with an increased risk of breast cancer, however these factors would not usually necessitate early or frequent mammography testing. Factors that increase the risk of breast cancer are:

- never having children or if your first child was born after you were 30 years of age

‘I went to a new GP for a general grease and oil change and she said it would be a good idea to have a mammogram as I was now 46 years old. I didn’t think much about being recalled for a second mammogram until they suggested I bring someone with me. It was an absolute shock being told I had cancer. I was thrown into the very foreign world of medicine and began living from one doctor’s appointment to the next. The hardest thing was telling my children and the best thing was the overwhelming kindness of people. I had an excellent result from surgery and radiotherapy. But there is no guarantee. People think it’s not going to happen to them, but it can. Breast screening with mammography is vital.’ Maria

- reaching menopause over the age of 55
- being above your healthy weight
- a history of excessive alcohol intake
- long-term use of postmenopausal hormone replacement therapy.

There is some evidence that breastfeeding may slightly lower breast cancer risk. Late onset of periods in adolescence and early menopause are also associated with a lower risk. This may be due to a reduced number of menstrual cycles.

RED ALERT!!!!

See your GP immediately if you notice:

- a lump, lumpiness or thickening in the breast or armpit
- changes in the skin of your breast—dimpling, puckering or redness
- changes in the nipple shape
- nipple discharge
- an area that feels different from the rest of your breast
- unusual pain.

What are the warning signs?

It is recommended that women of all ages be aware of how their breasts normally look and feel and report any new or unusual changes promptly to their GP. About 50 per cent of breast cancers are diagnosed after a lump is found by a woman or her doctor.

If you notice a breast lump, you must consult your GP immediately and have a biopsy to confirm the diagnosis.

How can you prevent breast cancer?

Exercise and a diet high in mono-unsaturated fat, vegetables and fruit may reduce the risk of breast cancer. Alcohol consumption increases the risk. However, many of the risk factors cannot be modified. Mastectomy is not usually recommended as a preventive measure in women with a strong family history or abnormal genes.

When to have a screening test

All women from the age of 50 to 69 should have a mammogram every two years. Mammograms are not recommended as routine screening of women younger than 40 as the test can be unreliable and ineffective. The tissue of younger women's breasts tends to be more dense due to the influence of hormones and therefore cancer will be more difficult to find. There is also some concern about exposing younger women to excessive amounts of radiation.

It is debatable whether women in the age group between 40 to 49 require routine mammography and the decision probably relates to personal choice and risk factors. Women 70 years and over may choose to continue having a mammogram. If in doubt, talk to your GP.

If you have one or two relatives diagnosed with breast cancer before the age of 50, or two first-degree (direct relative such as your mother, sister or daughter) or second-degree (your aunt or grandmother) relatives on the same side of the family diagnosed with breast or ovarian cancer or are at a higher risk of developing the disease, you may wish to consider genetic testing. Your doctor will recommend an individualised program, including more frequent and early mammograms if you have a very strong family history of breast cancer or test positive for BRCA 1 and 2 mutations on genetic screening.

What are the treatments?

Like most cancers, the survival rate for breast cancer is much improved with early diagnosis and treatment. Depending on the stage of the cancer, early treatment with surgery (excision of the lump or mastectomy), radiotherapy and chemotherapy can be very effective.

Detection of breast cancer while it is still small and confined to the breast provides the best chance of

TAKE AWAY MESSAGE

All women from the age of 50 should have a mammogram every two years. Mammography under 40 years of age is much less reliable and screening between 40 and 49 is up to the individual, based on risk factors. About 50 per cent of all breast cancers are found as breast lumps and all breast lumps should be biopsied, whatever your age. Breast lumps can now be more easily biopsied with a fine probe under local anaesthetic. Unfortunately many women fear cancer and disfiguring surgery and delay seeking a diagnosis. If you notice any changes in your breasts, consult your GP without delay.

effective surgery for women with the disease. Benefits of early detection include increased survival, increased treatment options and improved quality of life.

Over 70 per cent of cases of breast cancer are found in women aged over 50. However, in younger women tumours are likely to be larger and more aggressive and the overall survival rate is lower than for older women with the disease. It is therefore important that women of all ages understand that finding and treating breast cancer early is vital.

BOWEL CANCER

Bowel cancer occurs when abnormal cells in the lining of the bowel grow out of control, most commonly in the large bowel (the colon and the rectum). Bowel cancer is the fourth most common cancer in the world. Australia has one of the highest rates of bowel cancer in the world, and the rate is increasing. Bowel cancer is uncommon before the age of 40.

fast facts

There are over 12 000 new bowel cancers diagnosed every year. About 1 in 21 people will develop bowel cancer.

RISK QUIZ FOR BOWEL CANCER

DO YOU HAVE ANY OF THE FOLLOWING RISK FACTORS?		
Over 50	Yes	No
Personal history of bowel polyps	Yes	No
Familial polyposis (an inherited condition of multiple benign tumours in the bowel)	Yes	No
A family history of bowel cancer	Yes	No
Ulcerative colitis for more than eight years	Yes	No

If you answered 'Yes' to any question, consult your GP for advice on screening for bowel cancer.

Who is at risk?

There is a strong family link with bowel cancer. For example, anyone who has had a parent, child or brother and sister diagnosed with bowel cancer before the age of 55 years is at increased risk. This risk increases further if more relatives are affected.

How can you prevent bowel cancer?

A healthy lifestyle is an extremely important factor in preventing bowel cancer. Up to 70 per cent of cases can be prevented by choosing to eat well and exercise. The basics of a healthy lifestyle are physical activity and a diet high in vegetables and

'Very few people like to talk about their bowels. It's too embarrassing and we'd rather not even talk to the doctor. I just mentioned in passing to my doctor that I had noticed one drop of blood and some mucus in the toilet bowl once and fortunately she took it seriously. My cancer was diagnosed 15 years ago and I have no sign of recurrence today. I still have regular check-ups.' Natasha

RED ALERT!!!!

The most common symptoms of bowel cancer include:

- blood or mucus in the faeces
- an unexpected change in bowel habit (for example diarrhoea or constipation for no obvious reason)
- pain and/or swelling in the lower abdomen
- constant tiredness
- weakness and paleness.

fibre. High red meat intake (especially processed meat) and alcohol may increase the risk of bowel cancer so these should be consumed in moderation or avoided.

When to have a screening test

Screening by faecal occult blood testing (FOBT) every two years is recommended for all those aged over 50 years. Faecal occult blood testing is a test for blood in your stools. The test can be arranged through your GP. When there is a close family history of bowel cancer, a colonoscopy is recommended every five years from the age of 50 or from an age 10 years younger than the age when your family member was diagnosed with bowel cancer. For some people at very high risk, colonoscopy is recommended at an earlier age and more frequently.

What are the treatments?

Some early cancerous polyps or small tumours of the bowel may be completely excised under colonoscopy. Others require open abdominal surgery (excision of the tumour and surrounding bowel) and chemotherapy. If picked up early, bowel cancer can be cured or life expectancy prolonged.

TAKE AWAY MESSAGE

If you notice blood in your faeces or an unexplained change in your bowel habit, consult your GP without delay for further investigation. All Australians over 50 years of age should have a faecal occult blood test every two years. If you have a close relative with a history of bowel cancer, or other risk factors for bowel cancer, you may require screening colonoscopy. Early detection of bowel cancer usually means cure. Ask your GP at what age you should start having testing.

Physical activity and a diet high in vegetables and fibre are protective for bowel cancer, while a high red meat intake (especially processed meat) and alcohol may increase the risk.

SKIN CANCER

fast facts

Skin cancer is highly preventable, yet, Australians suffer the highest rates of skin cancer in the world. Fortunately many skin cancers are very treatable.

There are four types of skin cancer and each of these have a different appearance. They are all related to abnormal skin cells growing out of control. (Refer to <www.sunsmart.com.au> to view images of different types of skin cancer.)

'I thought I would rather risk skin cancer than be pale in summertime. Now that I have been diagnosed with melanoma, I know I was wrong.' Matt

RED ALERT!!!!

A new skin lesion or any change in a lesion on the skin could be a skin cancer. Moles or freckles that grow, change shape or colour, bleed or ulcerate, or new spots that appear should be treated with suspicion. Have your GP check out any unusual spots as soon as possible.

Basal cell carcinoma is the most common type of skin cancer and it usually appears as a small, slow-growing ulcer with a pearly white edge. In most cases it is curable and only rarely does this cancer spread throughout the body.

Bowen's disease is a superficial skin cancer that can develop into a squamous cell carcinoma if left untreated. They are usually small, red, scaly patches and are quite commonly found on the lower legs and feet.

Squamous cell carcinoma is the second most common form of skin cancer. It is usually a non tender, crusty bleeding ulcer. It most commonly occurs on the parts of your body exposed to sunlight. Squamous cell carcinoma may occasionally spread throughout the body.

Malignant melanomas are a less common but more dangerous skin cancer. Melanomas can occur on any part of your body and may spread throughout your body and cause death. It usually appears as a new brown, red or black spot which changes and grows in size quickly. Occasionally, existing moles may turn into melanomas. Nearly 9000 Australians are diagnosed with melanoma each year.

Who is at risk?

If you are over 30 and had sun damage to your skin when you were younger, you have a higher risk of skin cancer. However, skin cancer can also appear in adolescents and young adults with certain risk factors (see risk quiz on page 122).

How can you prevent skin cancer?

Cover up when ultraviolet light is strongest—between 10 am and 3 pm. Here are some tips for protecting yourself from UV sunlight:

- Wear a protective broad-brimmed hat, a shirt with a collar and long sleeves, and long pants or skirt.
- Wear densely woven cloth—hold your clothing up to the light; if you can see through the fabric, it will not protect you from sunlight.
- Shelter under canopies, umbrellas and trees when outdoors.
- When swimming, wear a wet suit and use UPF 40+ (ultraviolet protection factor for clothing) rash shirts, swim tops and body suits.
- Protect your eyes with wraparound sunglasses that conform to the Australian Sunglass Standard 1067, and carry an eye protection factor (EPF) rating of 10.
- Use sunscreens that comply with the current Australian and New Zealand standard on all sun-exposed areas of your skin—generously apply SPF30+ broad spectrum, water-resistant sunscreen on all exposed areas 15 minutes before going outdoors and reapply at least every two hours and after swimming.
- Mild sunburn, tanning and solariums should be avoided.

These recommendations should be implemented from early childhood.

Why prevent skin cancer?

Each year, around 1200 Australians die from what is an almost totally preventable disease.

When to have a screening test

Regular self-examination of your skin is recommended in everyone aged over 13 years.

RISK QUIZ FOR SKIN CANCER

DO YOU HAVE ANY OF THE FOLLOWING RISK FACTORS?		
Family history of skin cancer in first degree relative	Yes	No
Fair complexion	Yes	No
Tendency to burn rather than tan	Yes	No
The presence of freckles or multiple atypical lesions	Yes	No
Light eye colour	Yes	No
Light or red hair colour	Yes	No
Aged over 40 years	Yes	No
Presence of sun damage	Yes	No
Past history of skin cancer	Yes	No
Long-term exposure to sun and sunburn	Yes	No
High childhood exposure to UV light	Yes	No

People with the above characteristics are at increased risk of skin cancer and should have their skin screened by a GP or dermatologist from a young age.

See your GP immediately if you are in any doubt about any skin lesion. People at very high risk should have their skin examined by their GP or dermatologist every year.

What are the treatments for skin cancer?

Skin cancer may often be completely excised under a local anaesthetic, leaving a small scar. Occasionally a skin graft or wider excision is necessary. Superficial skin lesions may be treated with liquid nitrogen, photodynamic therapy or topical creams.

TAKE AWAY MESSAGE

Be vigilant about skin protection from a young age. This means covering up with densely woven clothing or sitting under the shade of a canopy, particularly when the sun is at its strongest, or wearing a 30+ skin block when this is not possible. Any changes in your skin should be checked immediately. Biopsies and excisions are usually minor but can be life saving.

CERVICAL CANCER

Cervical cancer starts as abnormal cells in the surface of the cervix.

fast facts

Cervical cancer is one of the most preventable and curable of all cancers. One in 101 Australian women will develop cervical cancer in their lifetime.

Who is at risk?

All women who have ever had sex, up to the age of 70, need to have regular Pap smears, including those who no longer have sex. The risk of cervical cancer increases with age.

'I recently lost my mother and had been neglecting my health. The last thing I thought I needed was a Pap smear. Luckily my GP reminded me the test was due when I went in for a sick leave certificate. My Pap smear showed some cancer cells which were easily treated at the gynaecologist's office. My mum would have wanted me to look after myself. Now I will face up to regular check-ups—they are really not that bad.' Shirley

RED ALERT!!!!

Vaginal bleeding after sexual intercourse, between periods or after menopause could indicate cervical cancer and should never be ignored.

RISK QUIZ FOR CERVICAL CANCER

DO YOU HAVE ANY OF THE FOLLOWING RISK FACTORS?		
Early age of first intercourse, earlier than age 16	Yes	No
Smoking	Yes	No
Multiple sexual partners	Yes	No
Genital human papilloma virus (HPV) or other sexually transmitted infections	Yes	No
Prior abnormal result such as 'cervical intraepithelial neoplasia'	Yes	No
A mother who was prescribed the anti-miscarriage drug diethylstilboestrol (DES) (daughters seem to be at greater risk)	Yes	No

If you answered 'Yes' to any of these questions, discuss your screening needs with your GP.

What are the warning signs?

Most women with abnormal cell changes or the early stages of cervical cancer don't have any symptoms at all. Occasionally, abnormal vaginal bleeding or abnormal vaginal discharge may be a sign of cervical cancer. Any abnormal vaginal bleeding, including bleeding after sex, should be checked by your GP.

How can you prevent cervical cancer?

Cervical cancer does not occur in women who have never had sexual intercourse. Avoidance of the risk factors above may be more realistic than abstaining from sex. To reduce risk of sexually transmitted infections, always use a condom during sexual intercourse. A vaccine against certain types of human papilloma virus (HPV) is available for women in

Australia. It is designed to prevent HPV infection and is therefore more effective in women before they become sexually active. Three injections are required over a six month period and it is unclear at this stage how long the immunity lasts. Pap smears will still be necessary for women who have been vaccinated.

Why treat cervical cancer early?

It is estimated that up to 90 per cent of the most common type of cervical cancer may be prevented if cell changes are detected and treated early. However, each year in Australia more than 1000 new cases of cervical cancer are diagnosed and over 200 women die from this disease.

When to have a screening test

All sexually active women should have their first Pap smear about a year or two after first having sex and continue every two years until the age of 70. Women who have any unusual symptoms, such as unexpected bleeding or discharge or pains, should see their doctor, even if their last Pap smear was normal.

It is debatable whether the high-tech version of the traditional cervical cancer check picks up more abnormalities than the conventional cheaper tests.

What are the treatments for a positive Pap smear?

The majority of low-grade abnormalities are due to human papilloma virus (HPV) infection and will settle without any treatment after about one year. Like the common cold, there is no medication that makes any difference to clearing the virus. Various tests are used to detect or treat cervical cancer if a Pap smear shows significant abnormalities. Some of these tests include:

- colposcopy—examines the vagina and cervix with a magnifying instrument to check for abnormalities
- punch or target biopsy—a small tissue sample taken from the cervix during a colposcopy
- cone biopsy—a larger tissue sample is removed from the cervix under anaesthetic.

You should have a repeat colposcopy and cervical cytology about four months after you have been treated for a high-grade lesion and follow up at 12 months with cervical cytology and HPV typing. Cervical cytology and HPV typing are then repeated annually until both tests are negative.

The release of a cervical cancer vaccine is an important step forward in preventing cervical cancer.

TAKE AWAY MESSAGE

Up to 85 per cent of women who develop cervical cancer have either never had a Pap smear or have not had one for over ten years. It's extremely important for women who have ever been sexually active to have a Pap smear every two years until the age of 70. Fortunately, cervical cancer is usually slow growing and preceded by precancerous changes. It remains one of the easiest cancers to treat successfully.

OTHER CANCERS

Oral cancer

Oral or mouth cancer begins in the lining of the mouth and the tongue. You are at increased risk if you are a smoker, heavy drinker or use tobacco products. If you have been exposed to excessive sunlight you are more likely to develop cancer of the lip.

Symptoms can include a lump, an ulcer that will not heal, bleeding, trouble swallowing, changes in speech, loose teeth and sore gums. Most oral cancer is cured if treated at an early stage. Unfortunately, many people do not consult their doctor until the disease is well advanced.

Testicular cancer

Cancer of the testis is more common in younger men between the age of 15 and 30 years but can affect men of any age. Men at high risk of testicular cancer include those with an undescended testis or a family history of testicular cancer. Symptoms include a lump in the testis, which can be painless or aching, or a feeling of heaviness in the scrotum. In most cases, testicular cancer is curable especially if detected at an early stage. Although there is insufficient evidence to recommend routine screening for testicular cancer, every man should be aware of what his testes normally feel like. If you find a lump or any other change in your testes, you should see your GP as soon as possible.

Ovarian cancer

Cancer of the ovary usually occurs in women over 40 years. The symptoms of ovarian cancer are usually vague. They may include abdominal discomfort, bowel disturbance, fatigue, urinary symptoms and pelvic discomfort or pain. Occasionally there is abnormal bleeding from the vagina not related to periods.

Ovarian cancer is often not diagnosed until it is advanced. If you have a family history of ovarian or breast cancer, you may be at increased risk and can be screened through genetic tests; however, currently routine genetic screening is not recommended.

Uterine cancer

Cancer of the uterus usually occurs in women over the age of 50 years. If you experience any bleeding after menopause you must be investigated for uterine cancer. Uterine cancer can also present as bleeding between periods or abdominal pain. There is no routine screening test for uterine cancer; however, it does have a high cure rate.

Lymphoma

Lymphoma is a cancer affecting the lymphatic system. The two types are Hodgkin's and non-Hodgkin's lymphoma. Symptoms include swelling of lymph nodes anywhere in the body but especially in the neck, armpit or groin, unexplained fever, or weight loss or sweating at night time. Again, there is no screening test for lymphoma, but any persistently swollen lymph gland should be biopsied to exclude lymphoma.

There are many other cancers which affect Australians. More details are available at the Cancer Council Australia website <www.cancer.org.au>. If you notice any abnormal symptoms or changes in your body, it is important to consult with your GP. Many cancers can be cured if diagnosed early.

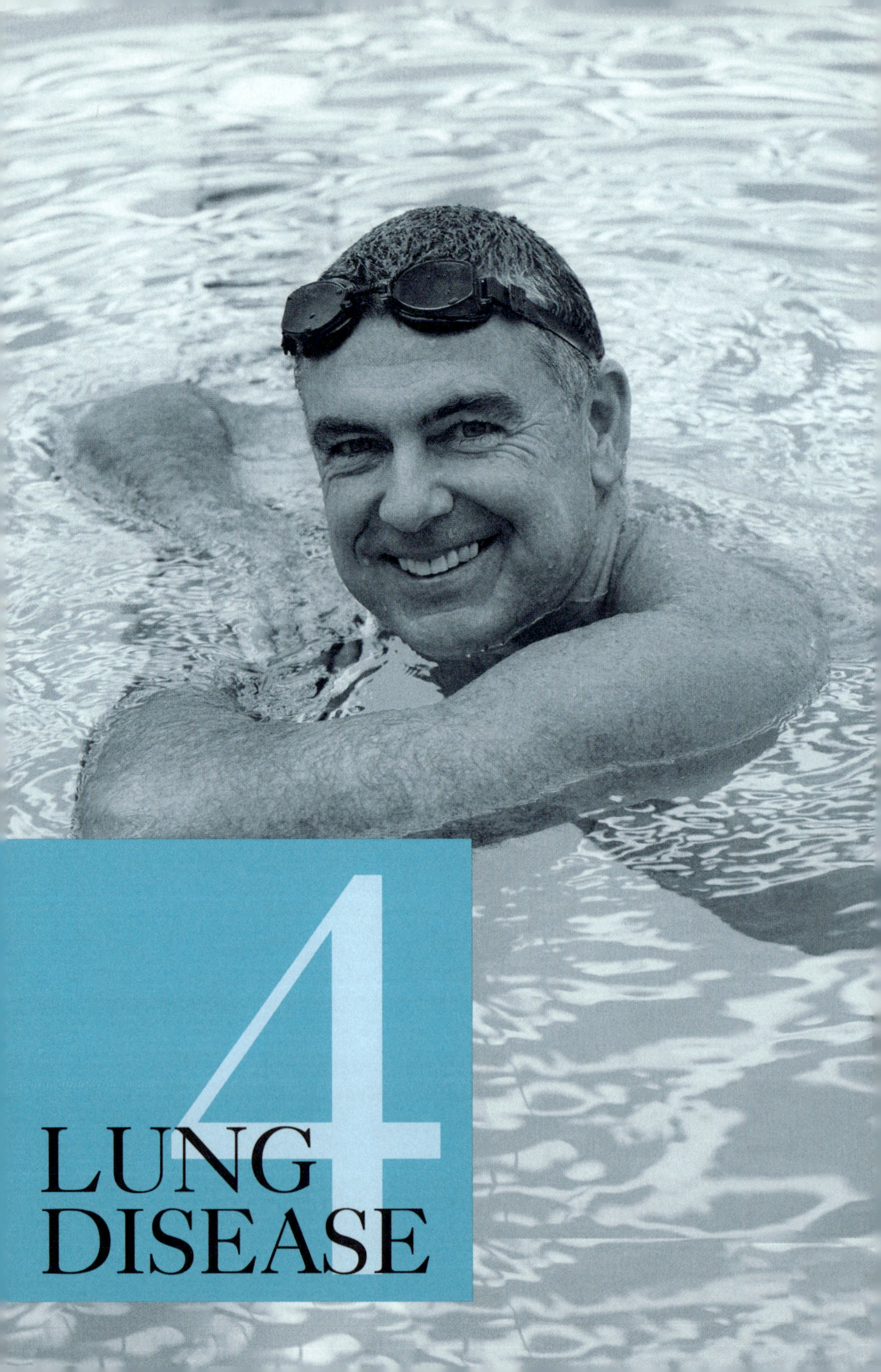

4 LUNG DISEASE

Lung disease

Asthma, chronic obstructive pulmonary disease and lung cancer are the most common causes of lung disorders and are often caused by smoking. Lung cancer is usually found at a late stage and can be difficult to treat. Asthma and chronic lung disease require aggressive treatment. Unfortunately, many Australians react to the breathlessness of lung disease by avoiding exercise instead of seeking effective treatment.

fast facts

The cost of respiratory diseases is about $3.7 billion per year.

What is asthma?

Asthma is reversible airways narrowing that occurs usually because of certain triggers such as viruses, cigarette smoke, exercise, allergen, dust, pollution, fire, a change in temperature, medication, a strong chemical, stress or particular food. Over two million Australians intermittently suffer the symptoms of asthma, which include dry cough (sometimes at night or early morning, or with exercise), chest tightness, shortness of breath and wheezing.

There are three main groups of asthma medications: preventers, relievers and symptom controllers. Preventers take a few weeks to reduce the redness, mucus and swelling and also reduce the risk

'There are times when I am extremely well but when I'm sick I'm really down. When I'm on cortisone, I sit up awake all night in a lounge chair because I can't stop coughing. I can only get half my words out from breathlessness and people can't understand me. I know I brought emphysema on myself from smoking. I didn't know it was harmful when I started—I thought it was a very glamorous thing to do. My message to younger smokers is, please don't smoke.' Hung

of asthma attacks and lung damage. Relievers provide immediate relief from asthma by relaxing the muscles in the airways. If you are using a reliever more than three times a week, it is a sign your asthma is not controlled and that you probably require a preventer. Symptom controllers are long-acting relievers, lasting up to 12 hours.

Your GP can help you develop an asthma plan to work out individual timing and dosage of your medications and how to respond to an asthma attack. A peak flow meter is a simple device to measure the condition of your asthma objectively. It helps predict when asthma is getting worse and whether the medication is correct. It's important to avoid triggers and to continue being active and to exercise. It's also important to clean your medication devices and to ensure that they have not expired.

Your personal asthma action plan will provide you with advice on how to know if your asthma is getting worse or is becoming severe or life threatening, and will provide you with directions on the use of medication at these times. If your asthma becomes life threatening you may have serious difficulty breathing or speaking, with little or no improvement with the use of your asthma inhaler. In this case, you should call for an ambulance on 000 or 112 if using a mobile telephone and state that you are having a serious asthma attack. Follow the directions of your asthma first aid plan. Keep taking four puffs of your reliever puffer every four minutes until the ambulance arrives.

RED ALERT!!!!

Signs of a severe asthma attack include gasping for breath, severe chest tightness, inability to speak more than one or two words each breath, feeling distressed, no improvement after using a reliever, and feeling pale and sweaty. An asthma attack is a medical emergency. Seek assistance and continue taking your reliever medication until you are able to receive urgent medical treatment.

What is chronic obstructive pulmonary disease or emphysema?

Chronic obstructive pulmonary disease or emphysema causes over 5200 deaths each year (3.9 per cent of all deaths) and is mostly due to tobacco smoking. About 490 000 Australians with this disease have chronic problems with mobility due to breathlessness and cough. If you cough several times each day, cough up mucus on most days, get more easily out of breath than other people your age and you are a smoker or ex-smoker, it is likely you have chronic obstructive pulmonary disease. Preventers, relievers and symptom controllers, as used for asthma, also improve the symptoms of this disease but they do not stop the decline in lung function. Antibiotics and oral steroids are sometimes required to prevent hospital admission; however, stopping smoking is your most important intervention.

What is lung cancer?

Primary lung cancer is a malignant tumour of the lung, where abnormal cells in the lining of the airways of your lungs grow out of control. It is the most common cause of death from cancer in Australia. Up to nine out of ten lung cancers are caused by smoking, including passive smoking. Once diagnosed, lung cancer often has a poor prognosis and it is usually not diagnosed soon enough to be cured.

Common symptoms of lung cancer are breathlessness, persistent cough, blood in phlegm or recurrent chest infections. There is no evidence that screening with chest X-rays reduces mortality from lung cancer and it is therefore not recommended.

Some lung cancers arise from abnormal cells in the lung itself. Other lung cancers are tumours that have spread from tumours in other parts of the body (secondary tumours). The ability to treat secondary tumours varies, depending on the type of primary cancer.

Immunisation for people at risk

If you have lung disease or smoke, you are more susceptible to 'flu (influenza) and pneumonia. In 2004, over 3000 Australians died from influenza and its complications. Each year there are about 650 serious cases of pneumococcal disease including pneumonia, meningitis and septicaemia, and nearly 100 deaths in Australians over 65 years of age.

Pneumococcal and 'flu vaccines are recommended for everyone over 65 years of age and also for younger people with asthma, diabetes, heart problems, kidney problems, pulmonary disease or other chronic illness, and for Aboriginal and Torres Strait Islander peoples and healthcare workers.

Tuberculosis

One of the most common causes of serious lung disease in the world is tuberculosis. Fortunately this is currently uncommon in Australia and immunisation and chest X-ray screening are no longer necessary. There are about 1000 new cases each year in Australia. People most at risk of tuberculosis include migrants and refugees from countries where tuberculosis is common and Aboriginal and Torres Strait Islander peoples living in the northern part of the country.

TAKE AWAY MESSAGE

Never ignore breathlessness, wheeze, persistent cough or blood-stained phlegm. They may be warning signs of lung disease or lung cancer, particularly if you smoke. Most cases of lung cancer and emphysema can be prevented by avoiding smoking. Asthma symptoms can be controlled by avoiding triggers and effective use of medication.

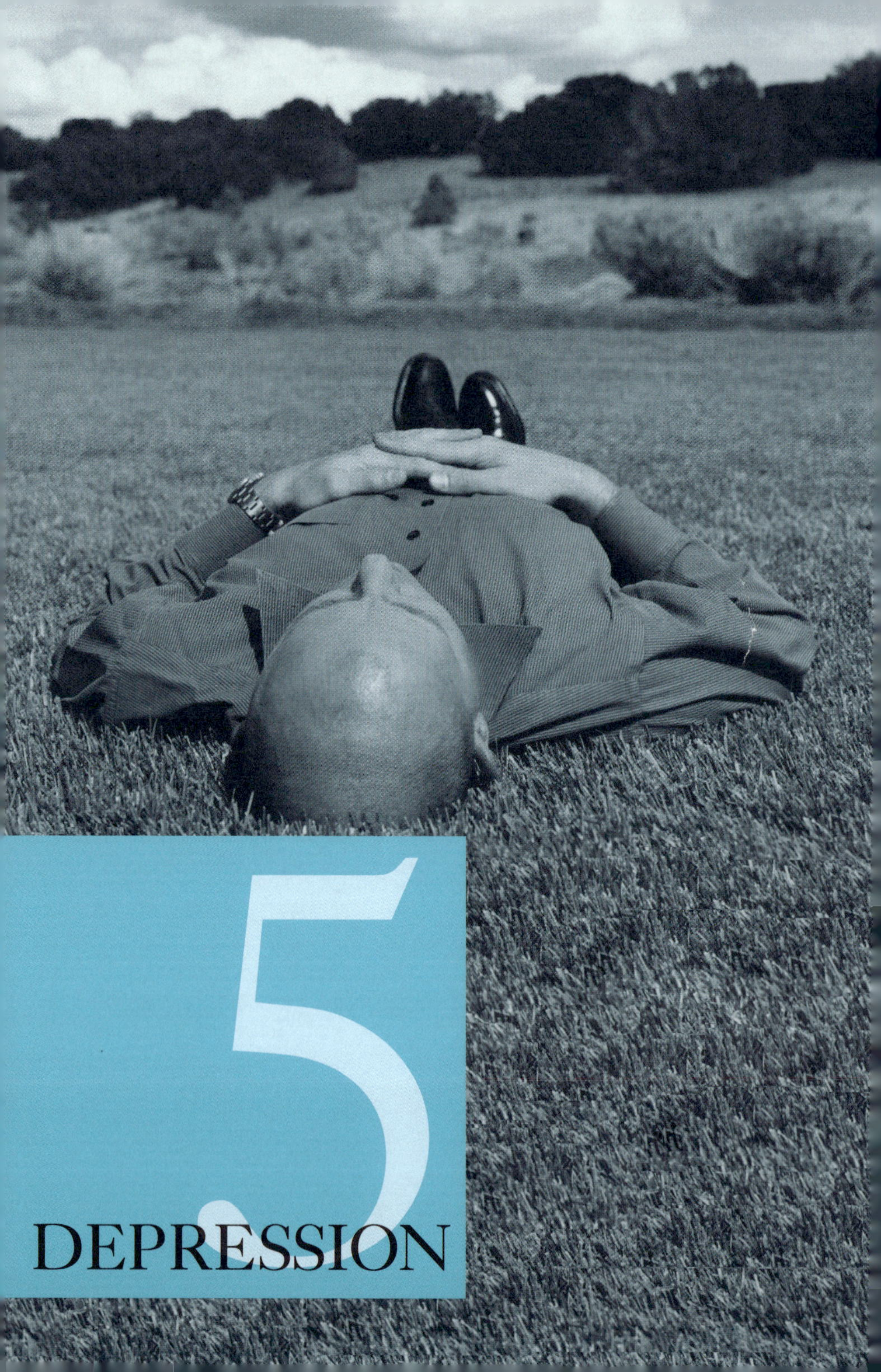

5 DEPRESSION

Depression

fast facts

Depression can be a killer. As well as adversely affecting your enjoyment of life, relationships and work, it is associated with suicide and with other physical illness including heart disease. About 20 per cent of Australians will experience depression at some stage of their lives.

'From my childhood I remember being unhappy. It was like a dark cloud descending on me. I remember my mother always being depressed. Despite all this, my life has gone well—I have a wonderful family and a good job. It was only when I accepted antidepressants that I felt the dark cloud finally lift. I can now think my way out of it. I am starting to feel a warm glow of happiness for the first time and I am not going back to that dark place again. I am only sorry that it took me so many years to express what I felt.' Sara

Unfortunately there is an enormous stigma against seeking help for depression and confusion over what depression is. Depression is a cluster of symptoms and may include sadness, irritability, disinterest in activities, change in weight and sleep patterns, restlessness, fatigue, feelings of worthlessness and guilt, poor concentration and sometimes thoughts of death. It's good to bear in mind that effective treatments are available.

What is depression?

Depression is much more than normal sadness. It is a cluster of symptoms that interferes with your ability to function. Irritability and relationship problems are sometimes more prominent than sad mood as indicators of depression.

About 20 per cent of people experience depression at some stage in their life. About 1.8 million Australians or 9.6 per cent of the population report having a mental health problem. The prevalence of mental illness is increasing and depression is predicted to become the second greatest cause of burden of disease by the year 2020.

Try this quick test to check whether you have depression.

DO YOU HAVE DEPRESSION?

DO YOU HAVE ANY OF THE FOLLOWING SYMPTOMS?		
Sad, down or miserable most of the time?	Yes	No
Loss of interest or pleasure in most of your usual activities?	Yes	No
Loss of or gained a lot of weight or a decrease or increase in appetite?	Yes	No
Sleep disturbance?	Yes	No
Slowed down, restless or excessively busy?	Yes	No
Tired or no energy?	Yes	No
Feelings of being worthless or guilty?	Yes	No
Poor concentration or difficulties thinking or indecision?	Yes	No
Loss of sex drive?	Yes	No
Negative thinking?	Yes	No
Generalised aches and pains?	Yes	No
Recurrent thoughts of death?	Yes	No

If you have two or more of these symptoms, we recommend you see your GP for further assessment.

Who is at risk?

It's important to remember that each person is different and it is often a combination of factors that puts a person at risk of depression.

RISK QUIZ FOR DEPRESSION

DO YOU HAVE ANY OF THE FOLLOWING RISK FACTORS?		
Past history of depression	Yes	No
Family history of depression	Yes	No
Excessive alcohol intake	Yes	No
Illicit drug use, including cannabis	Yes	No
Family conflict	Yes	No
Recent bereavement	Yes	No
Prolonged stress	Yes	No
Unemployment	Yes	No
Poor social support	Yes	No
Chronic illness	Yes	No
Certain personality factors, including a tendency to negative or perfectionist thinking	Yes	No

If you answered 'Yes' to any of the questions, you may be vulnerable to developing depression. Talk to your GP if in any doubt about whether you have depression as it is sometimes difficult to recognise it in yourself.

Depression robs people of the ability to enjoy life. Although suicide rates are falling, around 2000 Australians kill themselves each year. For every person who dies from suicide, at least another 30 people attempt suicide. Of those who have killed themselves, many have experienced depression or bipolar disorder. But many people who contemplate suicide but receive appropriate treatment for mental illness go on to lead productive, happy lives.

How can you prevent depression?

The key to preventing depression is in addressing some of your vulnerabilities, such as being a perfectionist, having negative thoughts, relationship difficulties, stress and drug abuse. (Ways to tackle stress and drug abuse are covered in more detail in Step 5.) Some practical strategies for protecting yourself against developing depression include challenging negative thinking, reviewing your goals and priorities regularly, relaxing more, improving your personal relationships, sleeping well, eating well, exercising and seeking help early.

Challenging negative thinking

If something is worrying you, firstly and most importantly, talk to a trusted member of your family or a friend. Think about what is important to you and look at your concerns with this in mind. Try doing the exercise on page 55 and identify your triggers for stress and helpful ways of releasing it.

If you find yourself thinking negative thoughts regularly, keep a daily diary of events that seem to trigger stress or a sad mood. You may be able to identify common unhelpful thinking patterns such as:

- automatic negative reactions—cynical, paranoic, perfectionistic, self-critical, expecting only the worst in people—to situations which set you up to respond negatively
- thinking black and white, awful or awesome, rather than seeing the more realistic touches of grey in life
- over-generalising, 'the everything always happens to me all of the time' attitude
- mind reading—sometimes your intuition about what others are thinking is wrong so try not to get down about what you think other people are thinking about you

RED ALERT!!!!

Depression has a major association with risk of suicide. Suicidal thinking is an emergency. Seek immediate attention from your local GP or mental health service if you or someone you know has expressed suicidal thoughts. The warning signs of suicide are:

- feelings of hopelessness, overwhelming guilt
- severe depression
- a sudden change in personality or strange behaviour
- insomnia
- unable to work
- no plans for the future

CONTINUED

- making a mountain out of a molehill, which means overreacting to things that don't seem to worry others
- wasting time worrying—focusing on things you can't change, while failing to focus on things you can do something about.

Challenge the evidence of your thinking in your mood diary. What supports your view? Are there other viewpoints? Is there another explanation or way of seeing things? What is the worst that could happen in this situation? What is the most realistic possibility? Is this thought helpful or unhelpful? What would I say to someone else if they asked my opinion?

These questions will help you break down a current problem into small parts:

- What effect is the problem having on my life?
- Imagine my problem has been solved, how would I feel?
- How would I know this had happened?
- What changes would I notice?
- What steps could I take to make these changes?
- What needs to change?

Identify things in your day which give you pleasure—simple, enjoyable things like playing sport, reading, breathing clean air, feeling the sun on your skin, talking to a friend, laughing, singing, taking a bath, listening to music, walking the dog, gardening, playing golf, going to the gym, swimming, cooking healthy food, riding a bike, learning another language, dancing, knitting, going to the theatre, reading a newspaper, taking photos, reading poetry, growing something from seed or fresh herbs on your windowsill. What are the simple things you enjoy?

RED ALERT!!!!

- admitting to feeling suicidal, written note
- expressing a plan for suicide
- giving away possessions
- unable to provide reassurance about safety
- feeling helpless, withdrawn, isolated.

Write them down and make time to do more of them every day.

Reviewing your goals and priorities regularly

It's only by reviewing your goals and priorities that you can create more balance in your life. If you are being overwhelmed, learn to say 'no' and manage your time by delegating appropriately and taking control of your life. Cut down on unnecessary work hours and find opportunities to enjoy life, eat well and exercise. Reduce your alcohol and coffee intake, and stop smoking, and taking any illegal drugs. (Refer to Step 5 for ideas on reducing risky behaviours.)

Identify at least two short- or long-term goals. These questions may help you do this:

- What things take up most of your time?
- Are there things you would like to be doing that you're not doing?
- What changes would you like to see in your life?
- What are your goals in the next few months (friends, family, work)?
- Where do you want to be in five to ten years?

Relaxing more

As discussed in Step 5, relaxation is very good for your mental and physical health. Simple techniques to increase mindfulness such as visualisation, muscular relaxation and breathing exercises work well. Practise letting go and 'watching' your thoughts. Imagine you are in a special place—the beach, a national park, your backyard, under your favourite tree—and allow your mind to experience the smells, noises, silence and colours of this imaginary inner world. Sit comfortably in a chair and progressively tense and then relax all your muscle groups, from your forehead to your fingertips and your toes. Close your eyes. Deep breathe in through your nose, hold for ten seconds and breathe out. Breathe in for three seconds, out for three seconds, repeatedly for one minute. Focus your attention on your breathing and counting—keep it smooth, expand your diaphragm on breath in and keep your chest still.

Improving your personal relationships

Better communication is the key to better personal relationships and resolving conflicts. If you have problems with communication, you are more likely to feel isolated. If you are isolated, you are more likely to feel depressed. As a first step in trying to improve communication, try 'active' listening in your next minor conflict with a friend or family member. Here are some of the features of active listening:

- Restate what you have heard from the other person in your own words, beginning your answer with phrases like, 'It sounds as if you think . . .' or, 'Let's see if I understand what you're saying . . .'.
- Try to be neutral in your answer and be aware of your body language.
- When you are ready to consider solving your differences, try to identify what's really behind the problem—what are you really trying to say?
- List all the possible solutions to the conflict and then choose the best solution together—if it does not work, try negotiating again.

At times of conflict, try beginning your response with statements like:

- 'If I understand you correctly, you think . . .'
- 'I see you don't understand what I'm saying, let me explain my rationale . . .'
- 'I see you are frustrated, let's talk about . . .'
- 'Blaming will not solve the problem, let's talk about how we can fix things . . .'
- 'I understand what you are saying and I would like to discuss another way of looking at things . . .'
- 'I am willing to discuss this with you when you are calm . . .'

Sleeping well

Problems with lack of sleep commonly precede depression and make fatigue and irritability worse. Avoid daytime or evening naps, time in bed without sleeping, inactivity (but don't exercise close to bedtime), work or stressful phone calls before bedtime, rethinking about today or tomorrow's stressful events, and drinks containing caffeine and alcohol.

To break the sleep/wake/insomnia cycle, only go to bed when sleepy. If you lay in bed awake for more than 30 minutes at any time of the night or early morning, get up and do something soothing—do this every time it happens throughout the night if necessary. Try to set yourself a routine time for getting up in the morning, no matter what time you went to bed or how tired you are. Stop lying there and worrying while in bed. Stop worrying that you cannot sleep. Try relaxation exercises and more physical exercise throughout the day instead.

Eating well

Some countries where people consume low amounts of fish oil tend to have a higher level of depression in their populations. This is supported by a number of studies, which also report some positive benefits on mental function of omega-3 fatty acids. In other studies, sugar avoidance has been found to relieve depression, while others have shown a short-term benefit in it lifting mood.

Heavy alcohol drinkers are more likely to suffer with depression. Caffeine has been found to increase mood swings and panic attacks in people with anxiety. As water makes up about 85 per cent of your brain weight, it makes sense to keep it adequately hydrated by drinking water rather than diuretics like cola and so-called energy drinks.

Eating fresh foods like nuts, seeds, fruits, dark leafy vegetables and wholegrain bread supports your brain function. Soy products are a great source of tryptophan, which is required for the production of the 'happy' hormone, serotonin.

Exercise

Exercise can be beneficial in assisting people with depression and anxiety. Refer to Step 4 for ideas on how to increase your daily exercise.

Seek help early

Unfortunately there is a lot of misinformation surrounding mental health and illness. Psychological therapies for stress and depression do work and antidepressant drug treatments can relieve the physical symptoms of depression. Do not hesitate to seek help from your GP or psychologist if you or a family member are feeling down or excessively irritable. It does help to talk about it and it can be life saving.

What are the treatments?

Depression can be treated. The most common treatment for depression is cognitive behavioural therapy, which challenges negative and distorted thinking. Your GP may refer you to a psychologist or psychiatrist for more specialised psychological counselling.

Newer antidepressant medication is very effective in adults and has fewer side effects than older medications. Despite some negative media and myths surrounding the newer class of drugs called 'selective serotonin reuptake inhibitors', they usually work well.

Your outlook is better if you seek help early and persevere with treatment for depression.

See the websites in Appendix 1 for those organisations that provide wonderful information about depression and other mental illnesses.

TAKE AWAY MESSAGE

Depression is a common and serious health risk. It is important to be proactive in protecting yourself against depression by challenging negative thinking, relaxing and exercising more, nurturing your personal relationships, sleeping and eating well, and seeking help early. Psychological counselling, cognitive behavioural therapy and antidepressant medications are all very effective treatments for depression.

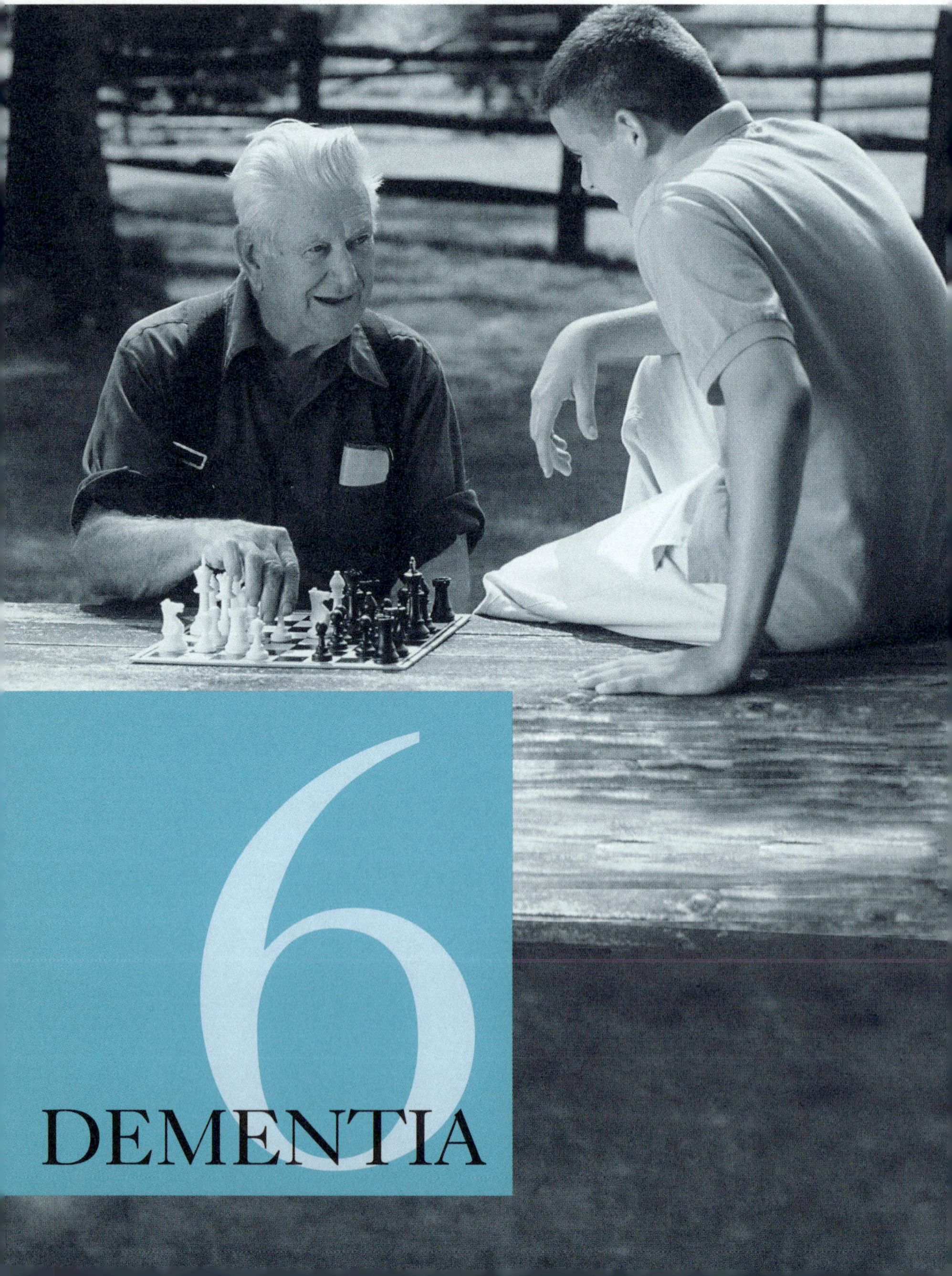

6 DEMENTIA

Dementia

fast facts

About one in fifteen Australians over the age of 65 have dementia. Some forms of dementia can be prevented and new drugs are available to treat dementia.

Dementia is the term used to describe the symptoms of a large group of illnesses that cause a progressive decline in a person's mental functioning. Most people with dementia are in the older age bracket, but it is important to remember that older people do not always get dementia. It is not a normal part of ageing. Dementia can happen in a person in their forties or fifties, but it is more common after the age of 65 years. However, people who complain of memory loss are more likely to have depression than dementia.

If you or someone you love has memory problems, seek help early. There may be important steps you can take to prevent or slow the deterioration of memory. Alzheimer's disease, vascular dementia and alcohol-related dementia are three common forms of this disease.

Alzheimer's disease is the most common form of dementia—accounting for between 50 and 70 per cent of all dementia cases—and is a progressive and eventually fatal disease of the brain.

> 'I know it's normal to forget things when you get older but I am terribly worried about Mother. She keeps leaving the gas on and the taps running. When you say something about it, she gets really upset. I am concerned she will hurt herself or someone else when she's driving.' Sam

The cause is unknown. Early symptoms include:

- memory loss
- vagueness
- taking longer to do routine tasks
- losing the point of a conversation.

Vascular dementia is the second most common cause of dementia and it is associated with problems in the circulation of blood to the brain, which cause a deterioration of mental abilities as a result of damaged areas in the brain. Vascular dementia may appear to be similar to Alzheimer's disease but like other strokes, it is preventable and treatable. (Refer to Chapter 2 on prevention and treatment of stroke.)

Alcohol-related dementia (Korsakoff's Syndrome) is another preventable form of dementia. Too much alcohol, particularly if associated with a diet deficient in thiamine (vitamin B1), can lead to irreversible brain damage. The most vulnerable parts of the brain are those used for memory, and for planning, organising and judgement, and social skills and balance. Taking thiamine appears to help prevent this condition and may also prevent further damage occurring. Once diagnosed, abstinence from alcohol is essential. Clearly avoidance of excessive alcohol intake is extremely important in preventing the disorder.

Who is at risk?

The cause of Alzheimer's disease is largely unknown —factors such as high cholesterol, inflammation of brain tissue and head injury are currently under investigation. The only known risk factor for Alzheimer's disease is family history. The chance of developing Alzheimer's disease increases as you get older. Some estimates suggest that about one quarter of people aged over 85 years have Alzheimer's disease.

What are the warning signs?

Many people experience occasional problems with memory, like forgetting meetings, names, words or where the keys are. This is normal. Persistent memory loss or forgetting things often is more worrying. For example, someone with dementia might do the cooking, then forget to serve the meal or even that they made it. Someone with dementia can become lost in their own street, forgetting how to get home. They may forget simple words and use inappropriate words and put things in inappropriate places. Tasks such as driving become impossible. Everyone becomes a little sad from time to time but people with dementia can experience severe mood swings and paranoia, and may become withdrawn or disinhibited.

Remember that many conditions have symptoms similar to dementia, so it is important not to assume that someone has dementia just because some of the symptoms are present. Strokes, depression, alcoholism, infections, thyroid disorders, nutritional deficiencies and brain tumours can all cause dementia-like symptoms. Many of these conditions can be treated. Consult your GP if in any doubt.

If you are having difficulties with your memory, your GP may ask you to undertake a mini mental state examination, which assesses your orientation in time and place, your short-term and long-term recall, your comprehension of language, and your perception, judgement and mood.

Dementia is a severe disability. It is a broad term that describes a loss of memory, intellect, rationality, social skills and normal emotional reactions.

How can you prevent dementia?

There is no cure and no way yet proven to prevent Alzheimer's disease from developing. Doing puzzles and quizzes, eating fish, exercising and avoiding fast food may help. There is some research evidence to show that moderate alcohol intake and exercise lowers the risk of developing Alzheimer's disease.

As already discussed, dementia due to stroke or excessive alcohol can be prevented. In addition, there are a number of conditions masquerading as dementia. By treating these conditions, the symptoms of memory impairment will often disappear. These conditions include:

- some vitamin and hormone deficiencies
- depression
- medication interactions or over-medication
- infections
- brain tumours.

It is essential that a medical diagnosis is obtained as soon as symptoms first appear to ensure that a treatable condition is diagnosed and treated correctly.

Can diet help?

It is interesting that dementia seems to be associated with the same risk factors as for heart disease and stroke. Reducing obesity and lowering cholesterol seem to offer the best hope for small improvements in mental function. Oily fish is recommended, as are poly- and mono-unsaturated fats in avocados, olives, nuts and seeds. The Mediterranean diet has been associated with a reduced risk of Alzheimer's disease. Antioxidants are recommended in the form of foods rather than supplements, and include:

- wholegrains
- tea (especially green)
- red wine (one to two glasses per day)
- fruit and vegetables, including prunes, raisins, blueberries, spinach, brussels sprouts, plums, broccoli, beetroot, avocado, oranges, red grapes, red capsicums, cherries, kiwi fruit, onion, corn, eggplant.

What are the treatments?

Medications called 'acetylcholinesterase inhibitors' are approved for the treatment of Alzheimer's disease, but no drugs have been found to halt or slow the progress of the disease.

People with Alzheimer's disease often also have depression and this should be treated accordingly. Early recognition of Alzheimer's disease allows better education and support for people with dementia and their families, initiation of community support and attention to other medical issues.

TAKE AWAY MESSAGE

Do not assume you have Alzheimer's disease if you have temporary lapses of memory. Look for another cause as it is essential a medical diagnosis is obtained at an early stage. Depression is a more common reason for memory loss. Consult your GP early if you are concerned about yourself or a family member or friend.

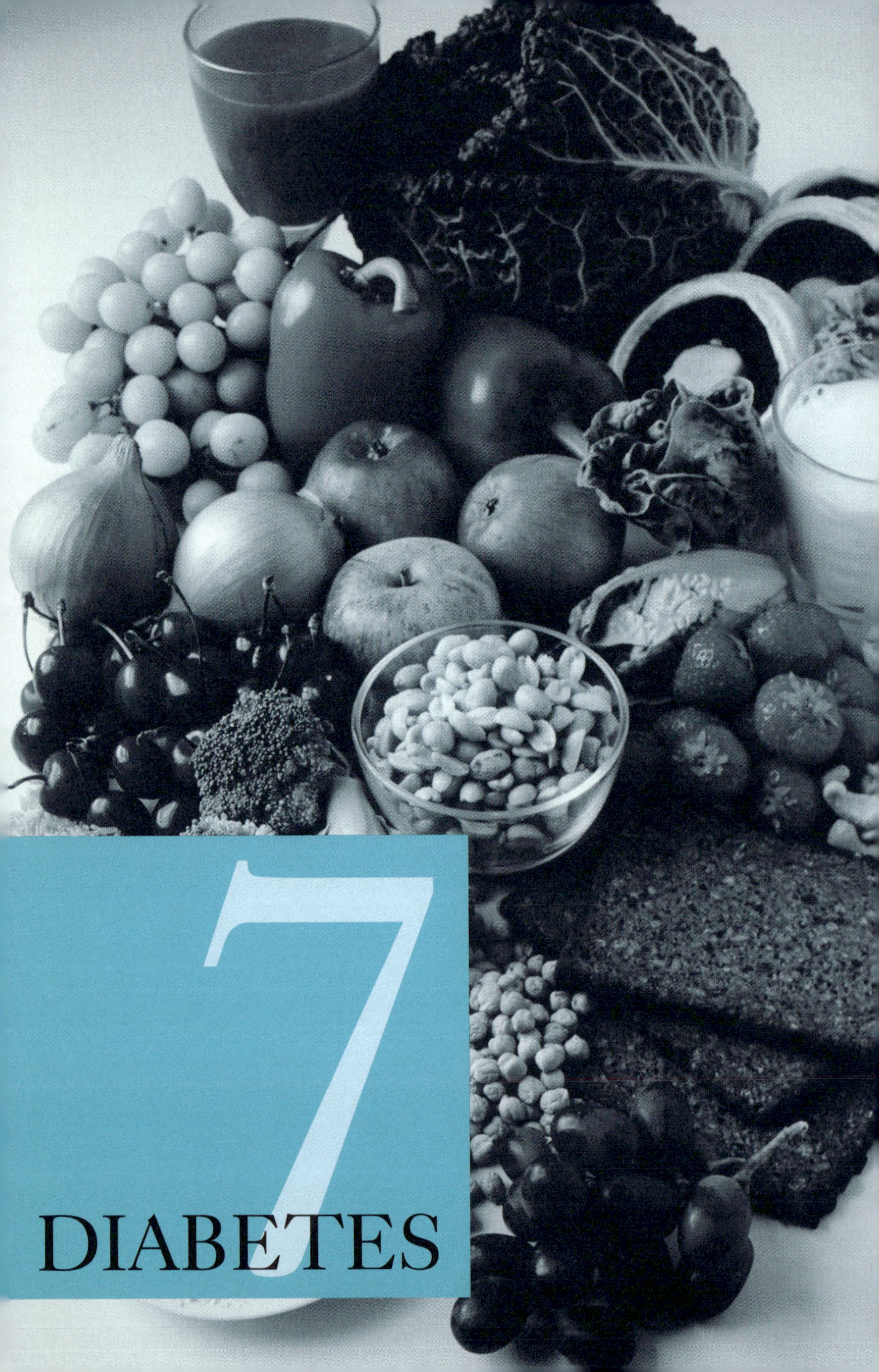

7 DIABETES

Diabetes

fast facts

There are about 500 000 people with undiagnosed diabetes in Australia, unknowingly developing irreversible complications. Of those who are diagnosed, only half are taking the correct amount of treatment. Are you one of them?

The prevalence of diabetes has more than doubled in the last ten years. Over 820 000 Australians now live with diabetes and approximately 12 000 die of diabetes complications each year.

Diabetes is a group of diseases characterised by high levels of blood glucose resulting from problems with insulin production and/or insulin action. Insulin is a hormone produced by the pancreas gland, which regulates glucose in the blood.

Type 2 diabetes is the most common form of diabetes and accounts for 90 per cent of cases. In this form of diabetes, cells of the body become more resistant to the action of insulin. Rates of type 2 diabetes have doubled in the last 20 years and are set to double again in the next 20 years.

Type 1 diabetes usually occurs in young age groups, and it is related to a lack of insulin and cannot be prevented.

The complications of diabetes include:

- premature death (twice as likely to die prematurely with diabetes)

‘My wife wanted me to go in for a prostate check now that I was 52 and overweight. My blood pressure was up and my blood sugar was high. My GP advised me about diet and to reduce my alcohol consumption. I now don’t eat junk food and watch my fat intake—simple changes really. My blood pressure has come down with one tablet a day.

My mother suffered from diabetes so I was aware of it. An associate had a check-up after what happened to me. He has been diagnosed with blood pressure and diabetes too. If I could go back ten years and cut down my alcohol and increase my exercise I could have prevented this. I had assumed bending and lifting at work as a mechanic would have been enough exercise. You’ve got to put in some more effort and be more conscious of what you eat.’ Jim

- heart disease
- stroke
- blindness
- kidney failure
- amputation
- impotence in men
- peripheral nerve problems
- bladder dysfunction.

Who is at risk?

RISK QUIZ FOR DIABETES

DO YOU HAVE ANY OF THE FOLLOWING RISK FACTORS?		
Family history of type 2 diabetes	Yes	No
Aboriginal and Torres Strait Islander background	Yes	No
Pacific Islander, Indian or Chinese background	Yes	No
Above healthy weight	Yes	No
Low physical activity	Yes	No
High blood pressure	Yes	No
Obstetric history of large babies or diabetes in pregnancy	Yes	No
Personal or family history of autoimmune disease (including over or under active thyroid)	Yes	No
Polycystic ovary syndrome	Yes	No
Personal or family history of heart disease or stroke	Yes	No
Smoking	Yes	No
High cholesterol	Yes	No

If you answered 'Yes' to any of these questions, you require a blood glucose test at a much younger age than your 55th birthday. Discuss your needs with your GP.

Everybody aged 55 and over should be screened with a fasting blood glucose every three years. There are many people with increased risks who need to be screened from an earlier age or more frequently as outlined in Step 1.

What are the warning signs?

You can have diabetes for years without being aware of it. Some specific signs include thirst and frequency of urine, including urinating at night. Other symptoms can include fatigue, altered vision and recurrent infections, including thrush and skin infections.

How can you prevent diabetes?

Prevention and treatment for diabetes centre around healthy eating, exercising and weight control. At least 30 minutes of moderate intensity physical activity on most, preferably all, days of the week is recommended.

Diet

Low glycaemic, high-fibre, carbohydrate foods such as wholegrain breads and cereals, vegetables and fruit provide most of our energy needs and are associated with a lower risk of diabetes. The glycaemic index (GI) of carbohydrate foods is determined by how quickly foods release glucose into the bloodstream. Low glycaemic index foods are preferred as they produce a lower and slower rise in blood glucose levels and more constant blood glucose levels between meals. High glycaemic index foods result in a rapid rise in the level of blood glucose, followed by a sharp drop, sugar craving and low energy (see page 161, Sources of Low GI foods).

People with diabetes require low glycaemic foods to stabilise the blood glucose. It also makes sense for healthy people to choose low glycaemic foods to reduce sugar craving and improve energy levels. However the GI has limitations and we should not replace fruit, vegetables and cereals with junk foods on the basis of glycaemic index. For example, the GI of some fruits, vegetables and cereals can be higher than unhealthy snack foods such as biscuits and cakes. Some packaged foods promoted as being low-GI may be high in fat and energy; for example, ice-cream. Always check the list of ingredients and the energy and fat (kilojoule) content of packaged foods.

What are the treatments?

Borderline diabetes can often be treated with healthy nutrition and increased exercise. People with diabetes are generally encouraged to eat mainly low glycaemic high-fibre carbohydrate foods such as wholegrain breads and cereals, vegetables and fruit, and to reduce their intake of fat, especially saturated fat.

Once the diagnosis of diabetes has been established, complications must be screened for on a regular basis and treated aggressively. You should work with your GP to develop an annual plan for care of your diabetes including eye, heart, kidney and neurological tests, and regular blood tests to monitor blood glucose. There are a number of advances in the treatment of complications of diabetes, including laser therapy for diabetic eye disease.

Daily low-dose aspirin should be considered in people with diabetes to prevent heart disease and stroke. Glucose lowering medications may be required if blood glucose levels remain high. These drugs need careful monitoring of blood glucose with a home testing device called a glucometer. Some people will require insulin therapy.

SOURCES OF LOW GI FOODS

- Dried peas and beans—kidney beans, haricot beans, chickpeas and baked beans.
- Bread, especially pumpernickel, heavy wholegrain and heavy fruit breads.
- Wholegrain cereals, such as rolled oats, untoasted muesli, barley bran, rice bran and oat bran.
- Most fruit, especially apples, pears, oranges, cherries, grapefruit, peaches, plums.
- Grains, such as barley, buckwheat and bulgur.
- Rice, especially basmati and doongara.
- Most vegetables except potato are low in carbohydrate and can be eaten freely. Examples of lower GI alternatives to potato are sweet potato, yam or corn.

Some examples of the GI rating of various carbohydrates include:

- Low GI (less than 55): soy products, beans, fruit, milk, grainy bread.
- Medium GI (55 to 70): orange juice, potatoes, cheese, pasta, chocolate.
- High GI (greater than 70): sugar, biscuits, corn chips, white bread, white rice, polenta.

Refer to ‹www.nutritionaustralia.org› for more information.

TAKE AWAY MESSAGE

Diabetes is a silent epidemic in our community with life threatening complications. It can be prevented by a healthy lifestyle. All healthy people 55 years and over must be screened with a fasting blood glucose test every three years. People who are at higher risk should be screened from the age of 45 or earlier.

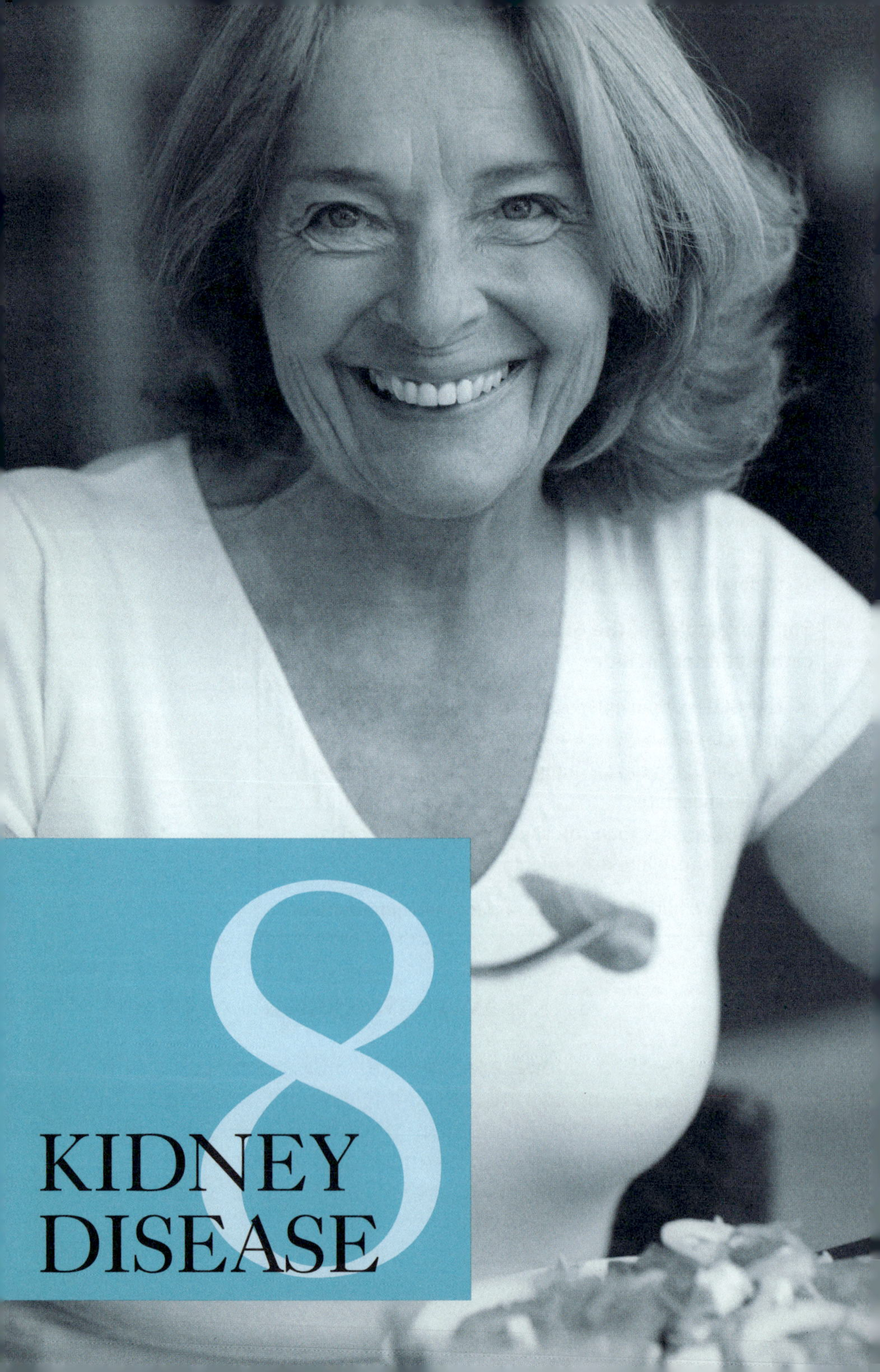

8 KIDNEY DISEASE

Kidney disease

fast facts

It is estimated that over 2.3 million Australians have signs of chronic kidney disease, including over 1.4 million people with moderate kidney failure. Eighty to 90 per cent of cases have not been diagnosed and unfortunately may only be recognised at a very late stage, when a kidney transplant is the only treatment option.

‘I’ve struggled with kidney disease since my early twenties. I had high blood pressure with my first pregnancy and then it never really went away. I have taken a lot of different blood pressure tablets and finally found some that suit me, but my kidneys have been permanently damaged over the years. I’m having dialysis and waiting for a kidney transplant. Except for being a bit tired, none of it has bothered me—it has bothered the doctors much more than me and now I know why.’ Emily

Chronic kidney disease is specifically kidney damage for over three months. Chronic kidney disease and failure are diagnosed by a blood test called a glomerular filtration rate (GFR). Up to 90 per cent of kidney function can be lost before there are outward signs or symptoms. One Australian dies of kidney disease every week waiting for a kidney transplant. The good news is that if kidney disease is recognised early it can usually be prevented from progressing, often with simple lifestyle changes.

Who is at risk?

Kidney disease may be related to a problem of the structure of the renal system present since birth or to chronic inflammation of the kidneys. Most commonly kidney disease is associated with lifestyle factors and genetic make up.

When should I have a screening test?

RISK QUIZ FOR KIDNEY DISEASE

DO YOU HAVE ANY OF THE FOLLOWING RISK FACTORS?		
High blood pressure	Yes	No
Diabetes	Yes	No
Aged over 50	Yes	No
Smoker	Yes	No
Family history of kidney disease	Yes	No
Aboriginal or Torres Strait Islander background	Yes	No

If you answered 'Yes' to any of the questions, consult your GP for a blood pressure and urine test even if you are younger than 50 years of age.

What are the warning signs?

Kidney disease often has few symptoms until it becomes very serious. Symptoms may include changes in the frequency of urination, blood in urine, pain in the back and swelling and puffiness of the ankles and face. As the kidneys fail, people may develop symptoms of tiredness, nausea, shortness of breath, loss of appetite and feeling generally unwell.

Kidney disease leads to high blood pressure, anaemia, malnutrition and heart disease, stroke and bone disorders. People with kidney disease are more likely to die of heart disease than to end up on dialysis.

If you are over 50 years of age, it is recommended you have your urine tested for protein every five years. Aboriginal or Torres Strait Islander peoples should be offered annual urine testing for protein from ages 15 to 18. People with high blood pressure, diabetes or a family history of kidney disease should also have an annual urinary microalbumin test, an annual blood test called a glomerular filtration rate, and annual measurement of their blood pressure.

How can you prevent kidney disease?

Treatment of high blood pressure, diabetes and high cholesterol, as well as weight reduction and quitting smoking, will prevent and treat many causes of kidney disease.

What are the treatments?

Once kidney disease is established, treatments involve dialysis, which is a process where the 'wastes' in the blood are removed artificially. In severe cases of kidney disease, kidney transplant may be the only option.

TAKE AWAY MESSAGE

The risk factors for kidney disease are the same as stroke and heart disease. If you are over 50 years of age, it is recommended you have your urine tested for protein every five years. If you have high blood pressure, diabetes or a family history of kidney disease, you should also have a urinary microalbumin test and a blood test called a glomerular filtration rate. Kidney disease is often silent and diagnosed late when it requires invasive treatments like dialysis and kidney transplant.

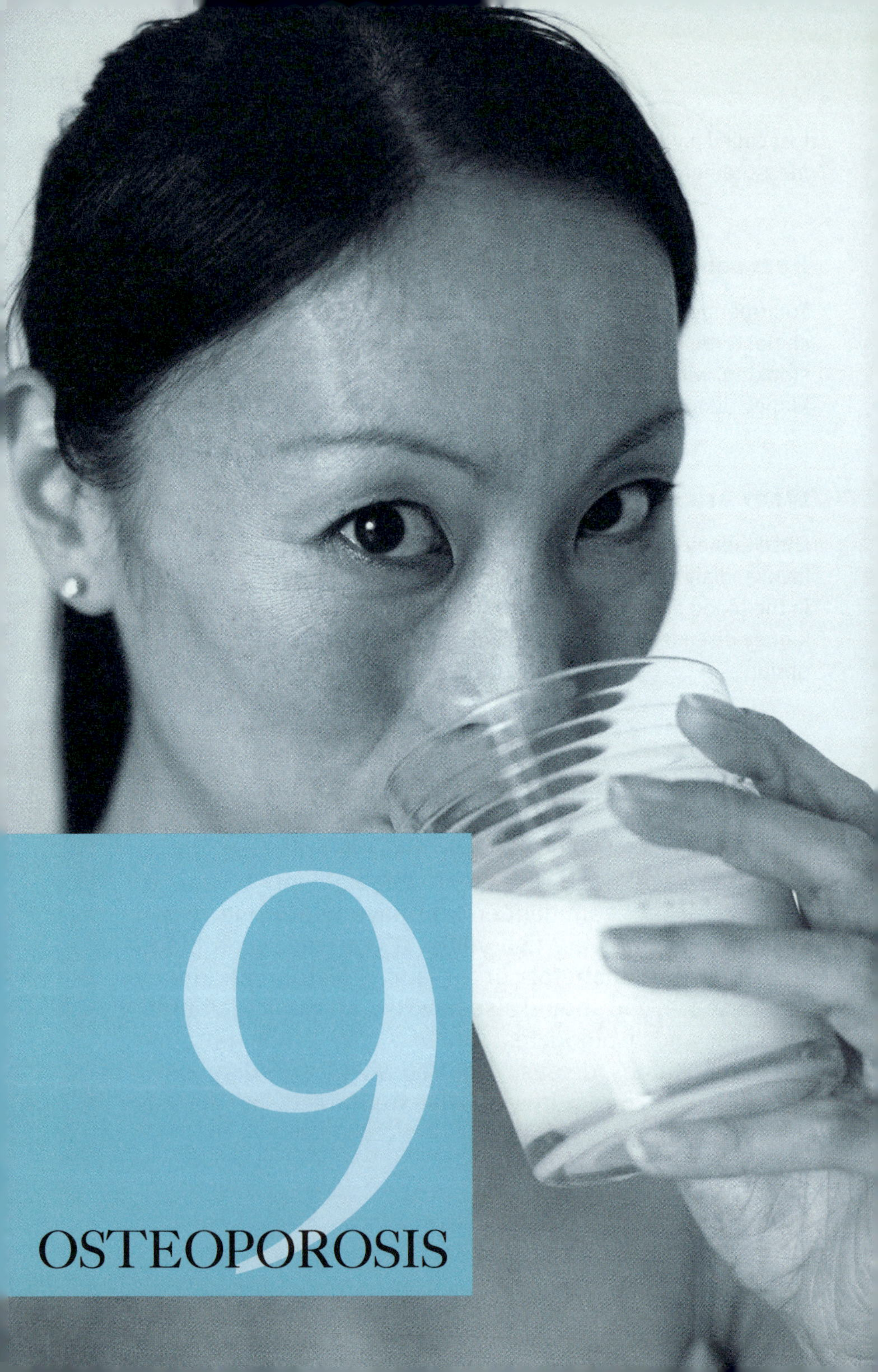

9
OSTEOPOROSIS

Osteoporosis

fast facts

About 2 million Australians have osteoporosis. Osteoporosis is common in both men and women.

Bone strength peaks at about 30 years of age and then declines, particularly in menopausal women. Osteoporosis is a condition in which the bones become more fragile and break more easily. It occurs when bones lose minerals such as calcium, and the body cannot replace these minerals fast enough to keep the bones healthy. As a result, bones become thinner and less dense. Any bone can be affected by osteoporosis, but the most common sites are the bones in your hip, spine, wrist, ribs, pelvis and upper arm.

Osteoporosis affects one in three women and one in five men over the age of 50 years. It is a major health problem in Australia, and studies around the country show that the incidence of fractures due to osteoporosis is increasing as our population ages. As many as four out of five people with osteoporosis don't know they have it, although they are at risk of fracturing a bone.

If you have osteoporosis or a history of fragility fractures or loss of spinal height, you need to take medication to prevent future fractures. The risk of death increases two to three times following an

‘At age 58 a masseur found a seriously sore point on my right hip. What got me thinking something was wrong was when the pain started to affect the way I played golf. An X-ray picked up signs of deterioration in the joint. I started taking pills for the pain. I considered a hip replacement—although the thought of such a big operation was scary. I've always been very active and now my life is back to normal. My mother and sister both had both hips replaced in their fifties. We all have osteoporosis and I take regular medication to help protect my left hip. I thought being a man I wouldn't go the way my mother has. She's now 89, with a severely bent over back and in full-time care. It's better to prevent these things.’ Marco

osteoporotic fracture so it is very surprising that only about 5 per cent of people who are eligible for treatment take medication to prevent further deterioration in osteoporosis or future fractures.

Who is at risk?

Many Australians do not understand the risk associated with osteoporosis and fail to exclude osteoporosis after a fracture or a joint replacement. A common late presentation of osteoporosis is the appearance of an obvious hunchback, and pain and disability. It is crucial that osteoporosis is diagnosed much earlier, before these symptoms appear, as it may be prevented by simple lifestyle measures alone.

As more bone is lost, fractures become increasingly likely. About two thirds of women over 60 years of age will have a fracture due to osteoporosis. It is important to prevent osteoporotic fractures by preventing and treating osteoporosis. Fractures can lead to long-term pain and disability, loss of independence, and may even contribute to premature death.

What are the warning signs?

Osteoporosis usually has no signs or symptoms until a fracture occurs, which is why it is often called a silent disease. Fractures due to osteoporosis are known as osteoporotic fractures. These can lead to changes in posture, muscle weakness, loss of height and deformity of the area affected. When the vertebrae are weakened they no longer support the weight of the body and become compressed, causing a hunchback and chronic back pain. In many cases, kyphosis or curvature of the spine is due to osteoporotic fractures of the spine.

No matter what your age, your bones should not break unless subjected to significant trauma. If you have a low trauma fracture, you may have osteoporosis and require treatment to prevent further bone loss.

RISK QUIZ FOR OSTEOPOROSIS

DO YOU HAVE ANY OF THE FOLLOWING RISK FACTORS?		
A women aged 45 and over or a man aged 50 and over	Yes	No
Low body weight (BMI less than 20)	Yes	No
Low or excessive physical activity	Yes	No
Family history of osteoporosis or hip fracture	Yes	No
Previous low trauma fracture	Yes	No
Certain medical conditions (e.g. chronic liver or renal disease, Crohn's disease, coeliac disease, thyroid disease)	Yes	No
Current or past history of taking prednisolone or cortisone	Yes	No
Eating disorder	Yes	No
Diet low in calcium	Yes	No
Lack of vitamin D (lack of sun exposure)	Yes	No
Smoking	Yes	No
Excessive alcohol intake	Yes	No
Menopause, if you are a woman, especially premature	Yes	No
Impotence, lack of libido or other symptoms related to low testosterone levels, if you are a man	Yes	No

If you answered 'Yes' to any of the questions, you may require an assessment to exclude osteoporosis. Discuss your options with your GP.

How can you prevent osteoporosis?

One of the best ways to build and maintain bones is by taking adequate calcium and vitamin D, and weight bearing or impact exercise such as walking, running, lifting weights, jumping or dancing. Back strengthening exercises reduce the chance of fracture by increasing bone support by the muscles. It is also important that you cease smoking, reduce your alcohol intake and prevent falls.

Diet

Calcium and vitamin D are essential to build healthy bones and prevent osteoporosis. The recommended daily intake of calcium is 800 to 1300 milligrams per day. While calcium is important for bones, it can also inhibit iron absorption. So try not to eat dairy products or take calcium supplements at the same time as eating iron-rich foods.

The highest sources of calcium are dairy products such as low-fat milk, yoghurt and cheese. Small amounts of calcium are found in breads, fruits, vegetables, cereals and fish such as salmon and sardines. Most people will receive their recommended daily intake of calcium by eating three serves of low-fat dairy products each day. If your diet does not include enough calcium, you may need a calcium supplement.

Vitamin D is ingested in the diet or formed in the skin through the action of ultraviolet light. Once it is absorbed into the liver it forms a compound that promotes absorption of calcium and phosphate from the bowel. A significant number of Australians are deficient in vitamin D because adequate vitamin D is unlikely to be received from diet alone. Vitamin D is found in oily fish (salmon, herring, sardines, trout, tuna and mackerel), liver, eggs, margarine and some low-fat milks. Exposure of your hands, face and arms to sunlight for about ten minutes in summer and about 30 minutes in winter, early in the morning or late in the afternoon is recommended to ensure you receive adequate vitamin D. If you have vitamin D deficiency you could take a supplement of 400IU of vitamin D per day. Your requirement for vitamin D increases as you get older.

When should I have a screening test?

All women aged 45 and over and all men aged 50 and over need assessment for risk factors for osteoporosis every 12 months. Risk factors include poor diet, limited sun exposure, loss of height, low trauma fracture and many medical conditions. At the same time, a GP may provide advice about modifying risks including a healthy diet, increase in physical activity, ceasing smoking and limiting alcohol and caffeine intake. Those with poor diet and limited sun exposure may be offered calcium and vitamin D supplements.

Osteoporosis is diagnosed with a bone densitometry test which is a safe, non-invasive special X-ray that takes about five minutes. People at high risk of osteoporosis should have a bone densitometry test every two years. This includes anyone 45 and over who sustains a low-trauma fracture and postmenopausal women with suspected spinal fracture or risk factors for osteoporosis. If you are 70 or over, you are eligible for bone densitometry. Medication is available on the Pharmaceutical Benefits Scheme for all people over 70 who have osteoporosis.

What are the treatments?

Your GP may recommend drug treatment to prevent further bone loss. There are a number of treatments available including:

- biphosphosphates which are effective treatments for fracture prevention
- selective oestrogen receptor modulators (SERMs), which are a first-line treatment for reduction of vertebral fractures in postmenopausal women
- hormone replacement therapy, which may be prescribed for postmenopausal women after reviewing associated risks such as cardiovascular disease, breast and uterine cancer and thrombosis.

TAKE AWAY MESSAGE

Adequate calcium and vitamin D intake is essential to prevent osteoporosis. You should be screened for osteoporosis from age 45 if you sustain a low-trauma fracture or have a vertebral fracture or other risk factors or specific medical conditions. Treatments for osteoporosis are very effective and can be life-saving.

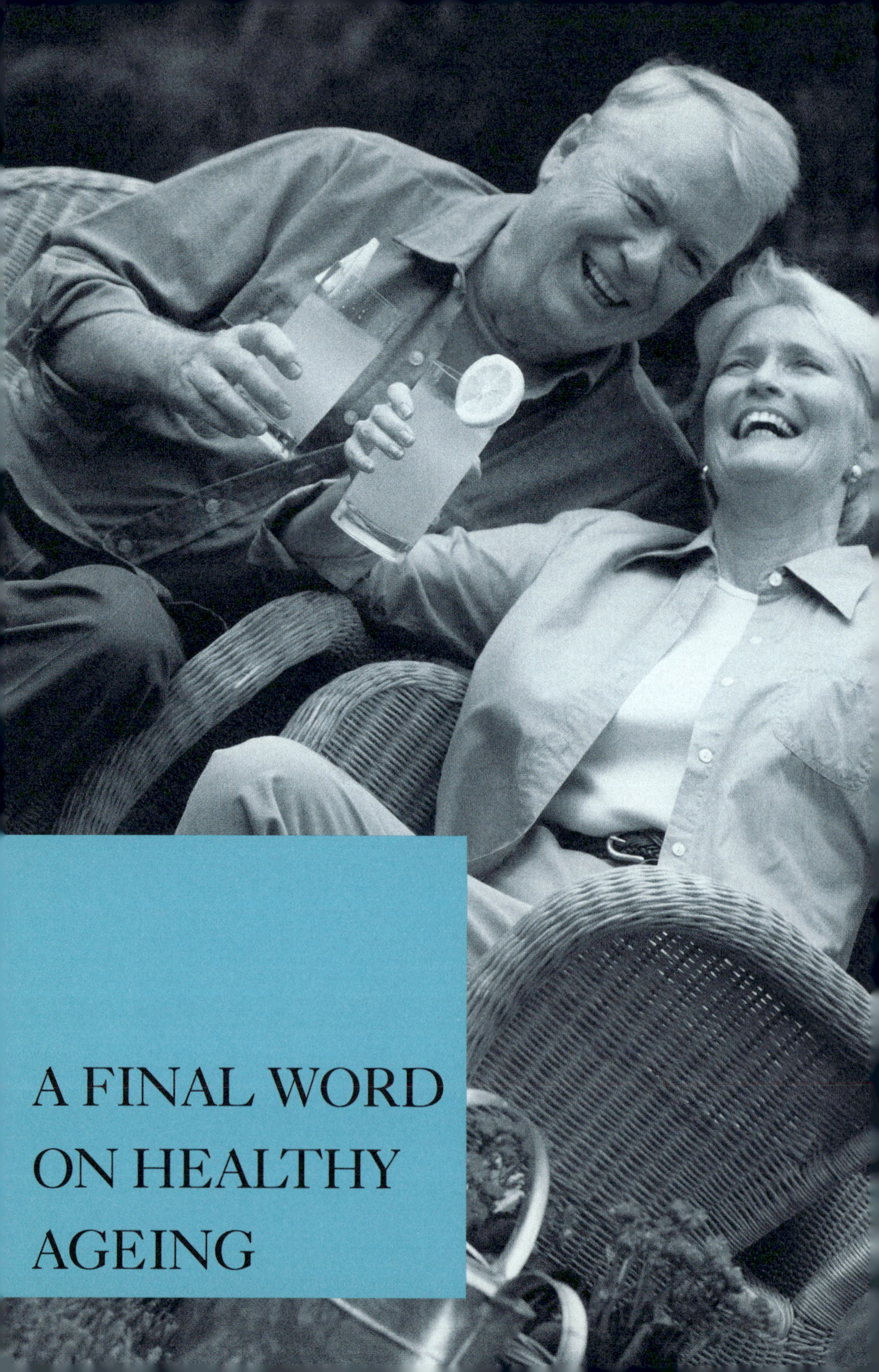

A FINAL WORD ON HEALTHY AGEING

A final word on healthy ageing

We hope that by following the recommendations in this book you will have a longer and healthier life. As you age further there are additional risks to your health.

Chronic pain

Although it is not a life threatening condition, which is the reason it has not been included in our book in detail, arthritis is the most common cause of chronic pain and disability. Contrary to popular belief, arthritis is not a form of natural ageing and many types of arthritis can be prevented and treated with activity, exercise and weight management. For more information refer to the Arthritis Australia website in Appendix 1, which provides detailed information about this important condition.

Falls

If you are aged 65 and over, you are at increased risk of falls which may lead to fractures and other serious injury. Falls are often related to balance problems, inactivity and reduced muscle strength. Discuss falls with your GP so that you can work together to ensure any medical problems are addressed and that your home environment is as safe as possible.

Visual and hearing impairment

Eye disease and vision impairment increase rapidly with each decade of life. Those at greatest risk of vision loss are older people, those with diabetes or a family history of vision impairment. Similarly, hearing impairment is common among those aged 65 years and over. As you age, have your hearing and vision tested regularly. This is particularly important if you continue to drive a motor vehicle. We recommend that everyone aged 50 to 64 years have their vision tested every five years and that everyone aged 65 years and over have their vision and hearing tested every 12 months. Aboriginal or Torres Strait Islander peoples require a vision check at least every two years from the age of 40 years. There are simple tests available for hearing and vision that your GP can carry out in the consulting room.

Medication issues

Older people are at increased risk of medication problems, particularly if they are taking multiple medicines. Medication error and interaction are common causes for hospital admission. Always bear in mind that the benefits of prescription drugs, non-prescription drugs and complementary medicines need to be weighed against their potential side effects and interactions.

When taking any prescription or non-prescription drug or complementary medicine, follow the instructions strictly and ask the following questions:

- Why is it needed?
- What are the side effects or interactions with other drugs?

- Are there better alternatives to taking medication?
- What will happen if I take nothing or forget the medication?
- How and when do I take this?

This information should be provided in the packaging of medications. If in doubt, ask your GP or pharmacist. Make sure your GP has a list of all the prescription, non-prescription and complementary medicine that you are taking.

We would all like to remain fit and healthy and active for as long as possible. Following our six steps on staying healthy, and being active in preventing and treating serious illness early, increase your chances of doing so. Some of what we have recommended may seem complex and challenging. This is where your own family doctor comes into the picture. Build on your partnership with your chosen GP to work together to keep you and those you love happy and healthy for as long as possible.

Appendix 1 Health websites

General health

www.healthinsite.gov.au
www.betterhealth.vic.gov.au

Alzheimer's disease

www.alzheimers.org.au (helpline on 1800 100 500)

Arthritis

www.arthritisaustralia.com.au (information on 1800 011 041, info@arthritisaustralia.com.au)

Asthma

www.nationalasthma.org.au (information on 1800 032 495, nac@NationalAsthma.org.au)

Australian Resuscitation Council

www.resus.org.au

Bowel Cancer

National Bowel Cancer Screening Program, www.cancerscreening.gov.au

Breast cancer

National Breast Cancer Centre, www.nbcc.org.au (information on 1800 624 973)
Breast Screen Australia, www.breastscreen.info.au (cancerscreening@health.gov.au)

Cancer

The Cancer Council of Australia, www.cancer.org.au (information on 13 11 20)

Cervical cancer

National Cervical Screening Program, www.cervicalscreen.health.gov.au/home (information on 13 15 56)

Depression

www.beyondblue.org.au (1300 224 636, for information on depression, anxiety and bipolar disorder)
www.ybblue.com.au (beyondblue's website for young people)
www.moodgym.anu.edu.au (cognitive behaviour therapy to prevent and treat depression)
www.bluepages.anu.edu.au (information on depression)
www.crufadclinic.org (information on depression and anxiety)
www.blackdoginstitute.org.au_(information about depression)

Diabetes

www.diabetesaustralia.com.au (information on 1300 136 588)

Dietitians (accredited)

www.daa.asn.au (information on 1800 812 942, nationaloffice@daa.asn.au)

Drug and alcohol information

www.adf.org.au (information on 03 9278 8100, adf@adf.org.au)

Genetic testing

www.genetics.com.au (information on 02 9926 7324, contact@genetics.com.au)

Healthy ageing

www.agedcareaustralia.gov.au

Heart disease

www.heartfoundation.com.au (Helpline: 1300 362 787)

Immunisation

www.immunise.health.gov.au (information on 1800 671 811)

Interpreters

Telephone Interpreter Service (13 14 50)

Kidney disease

www.kidney.org.au (information on 1800 4 543 639)

National Aboriginal Community Controlled Health Organisation

www.naccho.org.au

Nutrition

www.nutritionaustralia.org

Osteoporosis

www.osteoporosis.org.au (information on 1800 242 141)

Physical activity

www.healthyactive.gov.au

Preventive Health Guidelines of The Royal Australian College of General Practitioners

www.racgp.org.au/guidelines/redbook (guidelines for preventive activities in general practice)

www.racgp.org.au/guidelines/nationalguide (national guide to a preventive assessment in Aboriginal and Torres Strait Islander peoples

Prostate disease

www.prostate.org.au (information on 1800 220 099)

Safe sex

www.afao.org.au

Sexual health

www.shfpa.org.au
www.andrologyaustralia.org

Skin cancer

www.sunsmart.com.au

Smoking/Quitline

www.quitnow.info.au (helpline 13 18 48)

Sport and recreation organisations

www.ausport.gov.au
www.tams.act.gov.au/play/sport_and_recreation
www.dsr.nsw.gov.au
www.sportandrecreation.nt.gov.au
www.sportrec.qld.gov.au
www.recsport.sa.gov.au
www.development.tas.gov.au/sportrec
www.dpcd.vic.gov.au/sport

Stroke

www.strokefoundation.com.au (information on 1800 787 653)

Travel information

www.healthinsite.gov.au/topics/Travel_Health_and_Safety

Appendix 2 Adult immunisation

- A combined tetanus, diphtheria and pertussis (whooping cough) vaccine (dTpa) is recommended for everyone at 50 years of age who hasn't had a booster vaccine since age 17. A booster of dTpa is required for anyone with a tetanus-prone wound such as a wood splinter, burn, superficial wound contaminated with soil or manure, and if more than five years has lapsed since the last booster. It is no longer necessary to have ten yearly boosters of tetanus vaccine. The dTpa vaccine is also available with added booster protection against polio.

- Combined hepatitis A and B vaccine is available for people who are at risk of these illnesses including:

    - people travelling to areas of the world where the incidence of hepatitis A and B is high
    - medical, dental and nursing students and healthcare workers
    - men who have sex with men
    - people who inject drugs
    - people with chronic liver disease or people receiving certain blood products
    - staff and residents of homes for people with intellectual disability

  - people with haemophilia who may receive pooled plasma products.

- Free pneumococcal vaccine is available for everyone 65 years and over, as people in this age group are at higher risk of contracting life threatening pneumococcal pneumonia, septicaemia and meningitis than the rest of the population. A single booster is required five years after the first dose. Because Aboriginal and Torres Strait Islander people are also more at risk, free vaccination is available for all Indigenous people aged over 50 years and those aged 15 to 49 years who have medical risk factors. The risk factors include chronic illnesses such as compromised immune systems, HIV infection, kidney disease, diabetes, alcohol-related problems, heart or lung disease, asthma and smoking.

  Similarly, other people with chronic health problems under the age of 65 may benefit from pneumococcal vaccine and should discuss this with their GP.

- Annual influenza vaccination is free to people aged 65 and over as they are more likely to suffer complications from influenza. Each year a new strain of virus emerges in winter so the best time to be vaccinated is every autumn. It takes about two weeks to develop immunity. If you have an allergy to eggs, you should not be given influenza vaccine.

  Aboriginal and Torres Strait Islander people should be offered annual influenza vaccination from age 50 years or from age 6 months if they have chronic illness.

- Vaccination against human papilloma virus is available for women up to age 26, to help prevent cervical cancer.
- Vaccines are available for varicella (chickenpox), measles, mumps and rubella, for people who have not been previously immunised or exposed to these illnesses during childhood. Vaccines against meningococcal disease which can include meningitis, septicaemia and pneumonia is available for adults in Australia.

You can contact your state or territory health department for further information on the publicly funded vaccination program specific to your state or territory, or talk to your GP.

- Australian Capital Territory 02 6205 2300
- New South Wales Public Health Unit (there are several so look under 'Health' in the telephone directory for your nearest unit)
- Northern Territory 08 8922 8044
- Queensland 07 3234 1500
- South Australia 08 8226 7177
- Tasmania 1800 671 738
- Victoria 1300 882 008
- Western Australia 08 9321 1312

Appendix 3 Travel advice

Many Australians love to travel. You can visit the most exotic or remote locations on the planet and bump into fellow Australians. However, nothing spoils a holiday better than sickness and health problems.

If you have a chronic health problem it is a good idea to see your general practitioner for a check-up before you travel to ensure that you are fit enough to carry out your travel plans, to make sure that you have enough of your medications, and to ensure that you don't need any further tests before you leave. You don't want to risk having a heart attack in the middle of a trek through the Himalayas.

It is wise to take out travel insurance to cover any medical expenses or ambulance costs that may occur while you are overseas. The cost of bringing a seriously unwell or injured person back to Australia can be very high.

Remember to take all your medications with you. When you are flying it is better to pack them in your hand luggage rather than risk them going astray if your checked in luggage is lost, however you should consult with your airline as recent baggage restrictions may limit the amount of carry on luggage and especially the volume of any liquids and gels that can be carried on board. It is wise to travel with a letter from your general practitioner advising which medications you need to carry with you. It is also wise to travel with your medications in their original packaging with your name on the label.

Deep vein thrombosis (DVT) is a risk when travelling. A DVT is a blood clot that forms in the veins of your leg. If the clot breaks off it can travel to your lungs and cause blockage to the blood supply to your lungs. This can be fatal. There is considerable debate about whether sitting for prolonged periods on an aircraft can lead to an increased risk of DVT. Here are some recommendations to reduce the risk of DVT while travelling:

- Wear loose clothes.
- Drink plenty of fluids and avoid alcohol.
- Move about the cabin whenever you have the opportunity.
- Stretch your legs and feet while you are seated.
- Consult with your doctor before travelling about the use of graduated compression stockings or medication while flying.

Infectious diseases are a risk for travellers to many parts of the world. It is important that you consult your general practitioner or a reputable website for information on what you can do to avoid the infectious diseases which are present in the places you plan to visit. Many infectious diseases, such as malaria, cholera, typhoid, hepatitis, dengue fever, rabies, yellow fever and meningitis, can lead to serious illness and sometimes death. Simple measures include avoiding local water, taking care to only buy food which has been prepared under hygienic conditions, and avoiding being stung by mosquitoes.

Before you travel, especially to Asia, Africa, Central and South America and Pacific Islands, you should consult your general practitioner about whether you need any immunisations. You should do this a few months before you travel to allow any immunisations the time to be effective. Your general practitioner may also prescribe prophylactic medication to protect you from serious disease, such as malaria.

Some people engage in sexual activity while travelling. Remember that serious sexually transmitted infections such as HIV are more prevalent in many other parts of the world. Always practise safe sex.

One of the most common causes of serious health problems for Australians abroad is accidents, especially road traffic accidents. The road toll in many nations is much higher than in Australia and regulations on seat belts and speeding are sometimes much less stringent. Make sure that you always wear a seat belt, just as you would at home. Pedestrian accidents are also common. You need to take particular care when crossing the road in nations where cars are driven on the other side of the road as you may look the wrong way and then step out in front of a moving vehicle.

Travelling across time zones can have an impact on your body, leading to symptoms of jet lag. This can lead to fatigue, sleep disturbance, irritability, poor concentration and gastrointestinal upset. Getting plenty of sleep before and while travelling, and avoiding alcohol and heavy meals, can assist in reducing the symptoms of jet lag. Exposure to sunlight on arrival at your destination can also be beneficial. Give your body the chance to acclimatise when you travel across time zones.

Your general practitioner can be a great source of advice when you are planning your travel. Useful websites include the Better Health Channel (www.betterhealth.vic.gov.au) and the Australian Government HealthInsite (www.healthinsite.gov.au).

Index